The Last Season

A Compassionate End-of-Life Guide

Rebecca A. Brewer, RN BSN CHPN

Preface

Life is an amazing journey—a natural cycle of birth and death. These two profound moments are woven into the fabric of all our existence. While we often celebrate the joy of new beginnings, we seldom speak of the end, treating it as a silent knowing, afraid to look at it more deeply.

This guide is a gentle invitation to embrace the reality of life's last season, offering heartfelt guidance and support for end-of-life care. Whether standing by a loved one or reflecting on our own ending, this book aims to ease the transition and bring peace to these tender moments.

The process of dying is as unique as the individual experiencing it. It mirrors the essence of a person's life, be it with the quiet acceptance of serenity or the spirited resistance of a go-getter. At times, discomfort may arise and can be soothed, though some people's paths may present more challenges than others. In all circumstances, remember that we hold the reins of our journey. Speaking up about our needs, seeking the comfort we deserve, and asking the questions that weigh on our hearts are important. Crafting a thoughtful plan can be a

Preface

beacon of light during this final voyage. It provides a map into unfamiliar territory, which can be a source of soothing clarity.

May this guide serve as a compass and a companion, offering solace and understanding as we navigate the delicate dance of saying goodbye. As Ram Dass poignantly reminds us:

"We are all just walking each other home."

Chapter 1

Embracing the Conversation

"Death is not the opposite of life, but a part of it."

— Haruki Murakami

Engage fully in these end-of-life conversations with as much tenderness, compassion, and understanding as possible, yet also recognize the importance of the necessities. Facing the devastating reality of a loved one's or our own impending death is a profoundly challenging experience, accompanied by a flurry of fear, even terror, and many decisions. The initial shock and grief can feel overwhelming, making it difficult to navigate the necessary choices.

However, there is solace to be found in preparation. By acknowledging the situation, we can begin to organize and plan, making the journey as smooth as possible with the proper knowledge and support. This compassionate guide will provide invaluable insights and answer the many questions that arise, helping to regain a sense of control.

Encourage the person facing the end of life to participate in these decisions as much as they are able or want to. This involvement is crucial for their comfort and peace of mind and allows them (or us) to maintain a sense of dignity. Supporting their choices or our own ensures a more comfortable passing, surrounded by the people we wish to have close.

Talking about the end of life is one of the most emotional, profound, and challenging conversations we'll ever have. Often, we shy away from these discussions, not out of disinterest but because of fear, discomfort, or simply uncertainty about where to begin. However, avoiding these talks means missing the chance to hear someone's deepest wishes, which could ensure that their last chapter truly reflects who they are and what they value.

How to Start

We can begin by gently expressing our care and concern, saying something like, "I've been thinking a lot about the future, and I want to make sure we understand each other's wishes, no matter what happens." This acknowledges the gravity of the conversation while grounding it in love and concern.

Consider asking open-ended questions the other person can reflect on. For example, "What are your most important priorities if your health were to decline rapidly?" or "How do you feel about life support if recovery isn't possible?" These questions are about exploring wishes and allowing our loved ones to articulate what truly matters to them.

Active listening is just as important as asking. As our loved ones speak, we must listen actively, not just to the words but to the emotions behind them. We might say, "What are the things most important to you?" or "It sounds like you want to be comfortable at home with family." This kind of reflective listening ensures that we fully comprehend their wishes and shows that we're deeply engaged in what they're saying.

We can make the conversation even more meaningful by discussing specific scenarios. For example: "If you were unable to communicate, would you want aggressive treatments to extend your life, or would you prefer care focused on comfort?" Talking through these situations can provide concrete guidance for the future.

Last but not least, it's important to make sure these wishes are not just talked about but also documented. We could suggest, "Let's write down everything we've discussed so that everyone knows what you want." This ensures that their preferences are respected when the time comes and gives us all a sense of peace that the person's dying wishes are honored as they have dictated.

I can tell you that once the conversation begins, something remarkable happens—a sense of relief begins to settle in. By discussing death openly, we will realize it is also an opportunity to celebrate life and talk about our lives, and what we have accomplished and experienced together.

In these moments, we often uncover what truly matters most. Things we might not have known about each other can create a new intimacy. These conversations aren't just about filling out medical directives or deciding on a funeral service—they're a declaration: "This is how I want my final days to be," or "This is how I wish to be remembered."

It's also necessary to include practical details—like who will make decisions if they're unable to or what medical interventions (advanced directives) someone may want or not want.

Who will look after their pets, their home, or family keepsakes? These are crucial points that deserve thoughtful consideration. But for many, the more personal aspects hold the most importance.

If given the choice, how would we spend our last days? Would care be given at home, a family member's home, or a medical facility? Some people don't have the option of being in their own homes, so options for appropriate care are an important topic. These are intensely personal choices that deserve to be expressed and respected wherever possible. It is also important to recognize that it is not always possible. Being realistic about what kind of care and support is needed and what we, as caregivers, can provide is essential. Everyone deserves to leave this world in comfort and with dignity; these open and honest discussions will help us to achieve this for ourselves and our loved ones.

These discussions allow for decisions to be made by the individual, prior to when they may not be able to do so anymore. This is where advance directives, living wills, and healthcare proxies become invaluable. These documents ensure that people's wishes are respected and that the people they choose will be making sure that their wishes are carried out.

Advance Directives

Have open conversations about advance directives. This is one of the most important issues to talk about. Things to discuss include:

- **MOLST** (Medical Orders for Life-Sustaining Treatment)
- **DNR** (Do Not Resuscitate)
- **DNI** (Do Not Intubate)
- **DNH** (Do Not Hospitalize)

Such documents ensure that all wishes are carried out, even if someone can't speak for themselves any longer. By writing these choices down in advance, it also releases the burden on family members as well as healthcare providers when having to make tough decisions during a very emotional time.

At the end of life, discussing certain medical wishes, especially around life-saving measures, is common. For example, a DNR (Do Not Resuscitate) order means that if the person passes naturally or from their illness, no CPR or other life-saving actions will be taken. DNI (Do Not Intubate) means no breathing tubes will be inserted. There's also DNH, which stands for "Do Not Hospitalize," which is chosen when someone prefers not to go to the hospital for care. However, it doesn't mean they can't go if they have an unrelated injury, like a fall, that needs to be treated. In such cases, they might be treated and sent back home once stable.

Healthcare Proxy

A healthcare proxy is someone we entrust to make medical decisions on our behalf. Assigning this person can help reduce stress if tough or complex choices arise during end-of-life care. It's crucial to make sure all wishes are followed, and having a trusted person in charge can make that happen. Forms like 'Power of Attorney' and 'Living Wills' can be downloaded from different websites or obtained through doctors, healthcare providers, or social workers. It's important to have these plans in place well before any emergency arises. Pre-planning for things like burial or cremation and honoring religious or cultural rituals should also be part of this dialogue.

- **AARP Advance Directive Forms:** AARP provides free, state-specific forms for advance directives, including both Living Wills and Medical Powers of Attorney.

These documents are designed to comply with the legal requirements of each state, ensuring their validity. You can explore and download the forms at their official website: **AARP Advance Directive Forms**.

- **National Institute on Aging (NIA)**: The National Institute on Aging offers detailed guidance on advance care planning, which includes creating Living Wills and understanding the legal process. Although they do not provide specific forms for download, their website includes a wealth of information to guide you through creating these essential documents. Learn more at: **NIA Advance Care Planning**.

These resources are reliable and tailored to meet U.S. legal standards.

Emotional Anchors

Alongside the logistics of care that need to be addressed, there is, of course, the emotional rollercoaster this can set in motion.

Being with the People We Love

Family and Friends: In our final moments, being surrounded by the people we love makes all the difference. Whether it's holding someone's hand or sharing stories, those relationships can make us feel safe and less alone. It's finding comfort in knowing we've been loved and we've loved in return.

Legacy: Thinking about the ways we've touched others' lives gives us a sense of purpose. Even if it's something as simple as a conversation that changed someone's day, it's comforting to know we've left something good behind. Discuss this, and identify if there is something specific that the dying person wants to leave behind: a message, a lesson, or perhaps a journal with notes and keepsakes they have collected through their lifetime.

Spirituality and Faith

Belief in Something Bigger: For many, leaning on their faith during the end of life brings real peace. The idea of reuniting with loved ones, or simply trusting in a higher power, can make the journey feel less frightening. It's like having a guide into the unknown.

Traditions that Ground Us: Whether it's a prayer, a blessing, or lighting a candle, rituals give us something solid to hold on to. They're familiar and grounding, especially when everything else feels uncertain.

Finding Meaning: Even if we don't believe in anything religious, finding meaning in our life story or understanding our place in the circle of life can bring comfort. It's about knowing we matter.

Feeling in Control

Dignity in Choices: Being able to make choices even in our last stages—like where we spend our last days or what kind of care we wish to receive—gives us a sense of control. It's empowering to know we still have a say in how our story ends.

Finishing What We Started: Whether it's a last conversation, a final trip, or just tying up loose ends, being able to check things off our bucket list brings a sense of closure. It's like completing a chapter in a book—there's satisfaction in knowing we got to finish it.

Reflecting on Our Lives

Looking Back: As the end approaches, many of us feel the need to look back on our lives. Remembering the highs and lows, the people we loved, and the lessons we learned. Reminiscing and having good times together often evokes memories we will take with us in life and death. This is how we keep our loved ones with us as we have lived them together.

The Power of Presence

Simple Touches Matter: Sometimes, it's the simple things—holding someone's hand, a gentle touch, or just knowing someone is sitting beside us—that bring the most comfort. It's a reminder that we're not alone.

Being There Without Words: We don't always need to say the right thing. Sometimes, just being there—sitting in silence, listening, or simply offering a smile—means more than words ever could. Presence itself can be a powerful form of comfort.

Acceptance and Letting Go

Forgiveness: At the end of life, many of us feel the need to forgive or be forgiven. Letting go of old grudges and resentments or finally forgiving someone we've been hurt by can lift an enormous weight off our shoulders. It's about finding emotional closure.

Acceptance: Accepting that death is part of life, though hard, can bring a sense of peace. When we stop fighting against the inevitable and embrace it as part of the journey, it becomes less about fear and more about finding rest.

Love and Gratitude

Telling People We Love Them: Saying and expressing our love becomes one of the most important things as the end of our lives draws near. Whether it's through words, a note, a simple gesture, or simply saying "I love you," expressing love brings comfort and peace. It's a way of saying, "I'm here with you."

Gratitude for the Journey: Even with all the struggles, there's something powerful about reflecting on the good in life and feeling grateful for it. Focusing on what we've gained rather than what we're losing shifts the perspective and can make those final moments feel a little more peaceful.

Holding On to Hope

Hope for Peace: Even when there's no hope for recovery, we can still hold onto hope for release and peace—whether it's emotional, spiritual, or physical. The idea that—even in death—we can still allow hope brings comfort when the future feels so uncertain.

Living On Through Others: There's something deeply comforting about the idea that a part of us will continue to exist in the world, even after we're gone. Apart from our DNA that will live on in our children, there is the impact we made. It's not just about the grand gestures—sometimes it's as simple as knowing we've influenced others in small but meaningful ways. Maybe it's a kindness we showed, a lesson we taught, or even a passion we passed on. These little pieces of us live on in the people whose lives we've touched, and that can bring a sense of peace and purpose.

Hope for Transcendence: For many people, there's hope in believing that life doesn't truly end but continues in some way. A spiritual journey, reincarnation, a heaven, or even becoming part of the natural world. Whether we imagine our energy joining the universe or simply trust that our essence will remain in the hearts of those we love, this sense of transcendence can bring peace and a way to see beyond the limits of life as we know it.

For the Person Dying

Facing the Unknown

It is perfectly natural to feel afraid. What lies ahead is something none of us can fully predict nor comprehend. Doubts and fears can arise, like "Will it hurt?" or "How will it happen?" or "What changes can I expect?" All these questions can weigh heavy on our minds. But these thoughts will also help us start thinking about how we would like our last days, weeks, and months to be. It can be liberating to talk about these fears openly, learn what to expect, and seek comfort in cultural practices or through a trusted confidant. Facing these fears with honesty and support can bring a surprising sense of control to an otherwise uncontrollable situation.

Coping with Losing Independence

Adjusting to changes in our bodies, especially when it means losing some of our independence, can be one of the hardest things we need to face. It's tough to rely on others for things we've always managed on our own. This can conjure a mix of emotions—sadness, frustration, even anger and aggression. These feelings are perfectly natural and part of what's called anticipatory grief, where we start to process and mourn the changes happening. We need to give ourselves permission to feel all that we're feeling, practice self-love, and lean on friends, family, or spiritual support for encouragement.

Asking for help doesn't diminish our strength or who we are—it simply makes part of the journey easier. Focusing on what we can still control—whether making decisions about our care or finding small ways to maintain autonomy—can help greatly to navigate these challenges. Expressing our needs is instrumental.

Obviously, grief plays a big role in our last season and shows itself in various distinct stages—denial, anger, depression, bargaining, and eventually acceptance. But how we experience them is a very individual matter. So are spiritual comforts. I will go into much more detail on both these topics as we go.

For Loved Ones

Coping with the Stress of Caregiving

Taking on the role of caregiver can feel emotionally overwhelming. Especially if the roles are reversed, such as when we may be taking care of a parent, it's not just physically demanding; it can take a serious toll on our mental health and even strain relationships. It's important to remember that, as caregivers, we also need to look after ourselves. Throughout the book, and especially in Chapter 12, you will find a variety of self-care tips to help you cope in such emotional times.

Navigating Family Dynamics and Differences

End-of-life decisions can sometimes bring out different family opinions. "What's best?" "What would you want?" The conversations can lead to disagreements that might cause tension. In these final stages, the need for connection with loved ones may often become more intense. A person might want to hold on to those close to them a little tighter, spend more time with family members, share stories, laugh, and cry. This is a time to strengthen bonds. These intimate moments—whether spent in quiet reflection or deep conversation—are precious and can bring comfort and closeness to loved ones when needed most.

It is important, however, to understand that this is not always the case. There may be hard-to-handle choices that not everyone agrees with or is struggling to comprehend. Sometimes, the dying person may want to limit family, friends, or others' involvement or visitation. It is okay to set boundaries and advocate for our loved one's wishes in this regard. We don't owe people our time and should not feel bad when limits are enforced. An example of this is when family or friends might come for hours at a time just to feel more involved. This can be exhausting for the individual as well as for the caregiver. Limiting visits, creating an online schedule, or allowing people to drop by with meals, etc., is a great way to still involve those who want to help in a more controlled way. For more difficult situations, it is encouraged to seek support from a social worker, bereavement, or family counselor to navigate complex struggles.

The Moment of Letting Go

One of the hardest things to do at the end of life is letting go, letting the process happen. For many of us, the concept of people no longer eating food or taking fluids is daunting. These are usually the things we do as caregivers, the things we are taught to do, to make people feel better and more comfortable and to nurse them back to health. This is not what's required in the end; in fact, these things often don't help and can create discomfort. Sometimes, we continue holding on even when it is not what is best. It's important to understand that letting go doesn't mean giving up. Remember, this is about assisting in a comfortable transition, frequently reminding ourselves that these final moments are not about us, even as the spouse, child, friend, relative, or caregiver.

Honoring a Legacy

As we face the reality of our loved one's last moments, we might feel a strong urge to honor their memory. This could mean continuing family traditions, preserving their stories, or fulfilling any last wishes they've expressed. A task to discuss is to nominate someone who will write the obituary and establish important details that should be included to celebrate their life. Perhaps create a "life journal" to help us ask questions and start conversations with our loved ones and have a record of their life experiences. What are they proud of? What did they do for a career? What are they passionate about?

Walking This Path Together

- **Keep Talking:** Make sure to keep communication open and honest. Sharing our fears, hopes, and wishes and encouraging our family to do the same is a great way to stay connected, open, and supportive of each other.
- **Lean on Each Other:** Asking for help is never a weakness! A strong support system can provide comfort and help us process the emotions we're all going through. Take notice of yourself and others. Seek and give support when you see it is needed.
- **Cherish the time Together:** Spend time with the people we love. Shared stories and laughter, jokes, and lightheartedness can go a long way. Not everything has to be so serious all the time. Play favorite family games, watch movies, have a birthday party. As long as this fits the time and situation, don't be afraid to celebrate and be together.
- **Feel it all:** Allowing ourselves and our family to feel whatever emotions arise. Support and recognize each other's needs and encourage each other to express them.

Chapter 2

Care Options and Community Support

"Comfort comes not just from medicine, but from the presence of loved ones and the peace of mind knowing you are cared for."

— Kathy Kalina

Professional end-of-life care offers us various ways to ensure that a loved one is comfortable and has the support they need in their final days. Choosing the right option can feel incredibly difficult and overwhelming. It forces us to face reality, trying to honor care needs and wishes at the end of life. Hospice care, palliative care/bridge programs, and, alternatively, death doula support are all end-of-life care options. These services help navigate individual needs and the emotional challenges we encounter as we face the unknowns and the stress of watching and experiencing death. Let's explore some of the care options to consider and what services they offer.

Rebecca A. Brewer, RN BSN CHPN

Hospice Care: Compassionate Holistic Care

Death with dignity is a very basic definition of what the heart of hospice truly is about. The word "hospice" itself has become a trigger and creates fear in many people when, in fact, it comes from the word hospitality, which means to take care of. Hospice care can be given in most settings, including in the home, long-term care, nursing homes, assisted living, group homes, and even in rural areas and homeless situations when possible. Hospice meets the patient wherever they are. The only place a person cannot have hospice-level care is in an actual hospital.

CMO, or comfort measure, is often employed only when someone is in a hospital and is not able to go to another setting. Sometimes, people may be admitted as GIP (General In-Patient), as they may have pain or symptoms that could not be managed in another setting. This does not happen often but is sometimes necessary to ensure that care needs are met. Once the person is managed and comfortable, they are transferred back home or to an appropriate setting if possible.

Hospice care, however, is much more than just managing physical symptoms—it's a holistic approach that takes into account the emotional and spiritual needs of the dying person, as well as their family and caregivers. Hospice care is strongly encouraged to be sought out before increased needs or crises may occur. This gives the opportunity for relationships and trust to be established with the care team. They will be with us and support us even at night should we need it. Having this support early on will not hasten death but, in fact, promote quality of life.

It has been shown that having hospice at the end of life actually improves and extends life. The hospice team is called an interdisciplinary team, which includes a hospital medical director, nurse practitioners, nurse case managers, nurses' aides, social workers, chaplains, and spiritual support, as well as volunteers who work together to ensure this holistic support from all sides. Hospice can also help organize family care and local/community support. Many such programs offer comfort disciplines in the form of music, massages, and reiki.

The beauty of hospice support is centered on a "care surrounding" approach, helping patients and families to acclimatize and focus on the important things and ensuring measures are in place. Hospice is a covered Medicare benefit, and most commercial insurance plans cover hospice-level care.

Comfort measures: The hospice team will ensure that the patient is comfortable and free from suffering, discomfort, or pain. This may involve administering medications to ease anxiety, delirium, congestion, and shortness of breath. The aim is to allow the patient to pass peacefully and without distress. This also includes ensuring that they are clean and dry and repositioned frequently to prevent pain and skin breakdown. Providing frequent mouth care and soothing interventions such as music, massage, and spiritual practices.

Monitoring and support: The nurse case manager regularly checks on the patient depending on their needs for management. They will visit daily during the active dying phase to ensure comfort, pain, and symptom management. They are also available 24/7 on the phone and can make visits any time of day or night. There is a shift of focus away from close monitoring of vitals when death is imminent, as comfort is the goal. Other supports include SW, HHA, and Chaplain, all of which are available to help make this transition easier and to ensure that all patient and family/caregiver support needs are met. These disciplines work together for a peaceful passing.

Family involvement: Family members are encouraged to be present if that is the wish of the individual, as much as they want to be. The hospice and end-of-life team offers guidance on what to expect, helping us to stay informed about the process and what is happening, and providing emotional support and guidance. They might also facilitate important final conversations or moments of connection, need for closure, and bereavement assessment and support.

Palliative Care: More Comfort Alongside Treatment

Palliative care can be primary for symptom management with chronic pain and disease. However, when faced with end-of-life care, palliative care may play a different role as a bridge between seeking curative care and being able to transition, if needed, to hospice-level care.

Unlike hospice, which focuses on palliative and comfort at the end of life when there are no further curative options, palliative care can be started at any point during a serious illness. This level of care is there to help a person manage symptoms and improve their quality of life, even while they're still undergoing treatments and trying to achieve a cure.

Palliative care allows a person who is terminally ill to continue to seek curative treatments and have increased services as they are declining. Palliative-level care programs can serve as a smooth bridge to hospice-level care when and if it is needed. Very often, the hospice team is the same team as the palliative care team, which enables the continuity of nurses and other professional caregivers.

One of the best things about palliative care is its flexibility. It works alongside other treatments, which means a person doesn't have to choose between comfort or cure—they can have both. This approach allows someone to continue pursuing treatments if that's their choice while also focusing on what makes them feel better day-to-day. The goal is simple: to make sure they're living the best life possible, even in the face of serious illness. Palliative care is typically covered by most insurance plans and Medicare.

Palliative Care Focus

Comfort and symptom management: The primary focus is on alleviating any discomfort. Medications may be given to ease pain, manage breathlessness, bowels, or relieve anxiety. The care team continually monitors the patient to ensure they are comfortable and not in distress.

Support for the individual and family: The care team will offer additional support through nursing and personal care at home or even as an outpatient. They often have access to some of the services that are available through hospice, such as spiritual and social work support.

Time for a change: Sometimes, there needs to be a shift from palliative support to more intense hospice care. Palliative care very often helps to pave the way to end-of-life care in helping individuals and families come to terms with a loved one's decline while still having the support they need in place. This transition is not always achievable due to circumstances or the readiness of the individual. That being said, the palliative care and hospice teams can be mobilized quickly to ensure that care needs are adjusted and met accordingly.

Support Services for the End-of-Life Journey

Beyond hospice and palliative care, we can find many additional support services that will allow us to make the last months, weeks, and days of life more comfortable and less overwhelming.

Private care is another option that can be done in one's own home. If an agency is certified, it can usually administer and manage medications under the supervision of a nurse. These professionals provide one-to-one care, including overnight and 24/7 care. It's about bringing professional support right to someone's doorstep. Local options for personal care at home can often be found through the hospice and palliative care teams. They will have a list of acceptable providers in the area, as well as pricing. Private caregivers are hired for companionship and a presence for daily care and safety. They can be utilized in conjunction with other providers who may be coming in, such as the hospice home health aide. However, this is typically an out-of-pocket expense.

Doula service—or death doula—is another very personal touch that can make a big difference—it's about having someone around who understands what is needed and helps to maintain a person's dignity and independence as much as possible. Death doulas are professionals who provide non-medical care to a dying person. They are a wonderful resource for ensuring holistic needs are in place and end-of-life wishes are fulfilled. Unfortunately, this is also an out-of-pocket service.

Massages, music, and volunteering are provided by professionals who are trained and certified to administer their services. Volunteers help to provide a connection to the dying person. Very often, they are matched with someone with whom they have a commonality, such as a veteran or someone who has an artistic hobby. These services typically are offered through hospice care and are a part of the covered services. They do not have an out-of-pocket cost and are just for added comfort.

A wonderful story comes to mind of a lovely woman at the end of her life who was matched up with a good friend of mine. I had encouraged her to volunteer for the hospice I work for. My friend, a graphic designer, was paired with a woman who wished to write a book about being a Black woman living in the '60s. Together, they created a labor-of-love book, and she was able to help this woman fulfill her dream of writing it. Not only did they accomplish that, but they also touched each and every one of the hospice team members and friends who witnessed this endeavor. Her quality of life was absolutely improved by a hospice volunteer intervention, and her legacy and her story as well.

Tools and Resources

Making the Journey Easier: There are many tools and resources out there that can help us. These include web information forums, facebook, YouTube videos, or online and in-person support groups.

Compassion & Choices

- https://www.compassionandchoices.org/
- Offers tools for end-of-life planning, including advance directives, living wills, and palliative care resources.
- Online support through forums and guidance for making informed decisions regarding end-of-life care.

The Conversation Project

- https://theconversationproject.org/
- Free guides on how to have discussions about end-of-life wishes, including downloadable conversation starter kits.
- Tools for communicating with family members, caregivers, and healthcare professionals.

National Hospice and Palliative Care Organization (NHPCO)

- https://www.nhpco.org/
- Offers comprehensive information on hospice and palliative care services, as well as links to state-specific advance directive forms.

- Directory of local hospice and palliative care programs, with both in-person and virtual support groups.

Death Café

- https://deathcafe.com/
- An international platform where people gather (in-person or virtually) to discuss death and end-of-life topics in a supportive environment.
- Offers forums for open and respectful discussions on end-of-life topics. We can find local or online meetings.

End With Care

- https://endwithcare.org/
- Provides information on hospice care, grief support, and practical guides for planning end-of-life care.
- Includes listings of community-based end-of-life services and caregiver resources.

Facebook Groups (Online Support)

- **End-of-Life Discussion Group:** A space for people to discuss end-of-life care, share experiences, and find support.
- **Grief & Loss Support Group:** For individuals dealing with the loss of a loved one, this group offers emotional support and advice on navigating grief.
- **Palliative Care Community:** Provides educational resources and emotional support for those providing or receiving palliative care.

YouTube Channels (Educational Videos)

- **What Matters Most:** Focuses on personal stories, caregiver experiences, and professional advice on end-of-life care.
- **Death Positive Movement:** Channels like "Ask a Mortician" or "The Order of the Good Death" cover death, dying, and funerary practices in a compassionate, educational way.
- **Hospice Basics:** Offers videos that explain various aspects of hospice care, advance directives, and how to navigate end-of-life decisions.

Aging with Dignity (Five Wishes)

- **Website:** https://www.fivewishes.org/
- **Resources:** Provides a simple legal document that helps people specify how they want to be cared for at the end of their life.
- **Support:** Includes downloadable forms for advance care planning and end-of-life care preferences.

CaringInfo (NHPCO)

- **Website:** https://www.caringinfo.org/
- Provides free advance directives and planning guides specific to each state, as well as tips for caregivers and family members. Offers toll-free helpline and online support resources.

In-Person and Online Support Groups

- **Meetup:** Check for local or virtual end-of-life and grief support groups in our area via Meetup.
- **Hospice Organizations:** Many local hospices offer support groups for caregivers, families, and those

facing terminal illnesses. Check our local hospice for group meetings or virtual events.

These resources offer a combination of educational materials, legal tools, and community-driven discussions to help us and families navigate through such emotional times.

Looking up video tutorials can be especially helpful to find practical advice on things like:

- Bed-bound care
- Wound dressing
- Incontinence care
- How to Ffed someone
- Dementia care
- Administration of medication and ways to manage many medications and schedules.

Community and Other Support Groups

Both in-person and online support groups can be infinitely helpful in not only providing an additional support layer but also a place to ask questions and share experiences of end-of-life care, tips, and suggestions to make care easier. These groups offer a safe space to seek advice and find comfort in knowing that we're not alone. Connecting with others who are going through similar experiences can provide a sense of community and understanding that's incredibly valuable during this time.

Here are more website resources you may find useful:

- GetPalliativeCare.org
- https://hospicefoundation.org/
- https://www.nhpco.org/

- https://theconversationproject.org/
- https://deathwithdignity.org/

Chapter 3

Navigating Expectations and Needs: Care at Home

"Caring for others is the highest expression of humanity."

— Harriet Beecher Stowe

The profound and challenging journey we will find ourselves on when caring for a loved one is something we may not be sure we can provide. When we decide to provide care at home, it's essential to approach it with compassion and realistic expectations. Working in hospice and home care, I've seen firsthand the dedication families bring to this task. Of course, the desire to care for a loved one is a wonderful sentiment, but it's important to recognize the demands and limitations that can come with it and to realistically examine what we are capable of and can safely provide.

If our loved one is bedridden, providing care involves more than just being there. We'll be responsible for managing their comfort, administering medications, and taking care of personal needs like toileting, incontinence care, and bathing. These tasks, though manageable, can be physically demanding and emotionally exhausting.

Take, for example, assisting with toileting and maintaining hygiene. This is not just about cleanliness; it's about preserving someone's dignity during such tasks as they may feel very vulnerable and exposed.

As this is not an easy undertaking, it's perfectly okay to admit if you're struggling—it doesn't mean you care any less. Ask for help early on if you need it, and make sure you're looking after yourself, too.

Providing Realistic Care

In these final stages, the person you're caring for can often lose their ability to maintain their routine themselves, which can be heartbreaking to witness. Their vulnerability requires a lot of tenderness, patience, and emotional understanding.

Take an honest look at what you can realistically manage at home, taking all family members into consideration, too. This involves assessing not just your physical strength but also your emotional stamina. The nature of your loved one's illness plays a big role in determining whether home care is feasible or if more specialized care is a better option. In the final stages of their life, the level of care required increases, and what you could once handle alone may become too much.Obtaining additional support or transition to hospice care is strongly suggested to get the help you will need in order to navigate the challenges of providing good care. You will need to evaluate and re-evaluate what works and what doesn't and adjust accordingly.

Dependent and Bed-Bound Care Needs

Let's dive into what kind of care may be required at the end of life.

Skincare: For a bed-bound individual, the care routine becomes more specialized. Preventing bedsores is a major concern, as these can develop quickly and cause significant discomfort. Regularly turning and repositioning every 2-3 hours while in bed is key to preventing skin damage and breakdown. Keeping sheets wrinkle-free and obtaining a low air loss or specialty mattress to protect the skin is also very important. It does not take a lot of pressure to create a bed sore. Check skin regularly for redness and areas of breakdown or excoriation, including feet/heels, elbows, personal areas, back of the legs, and head. The use of barrier creams and protective dressings is also helpful in preserving and protecting skin integrity. If there is great discomfort with movement and personal care, discuss pre-medicating with your hospice team to ensure comfort is maintained.

Oral care: As eating and drinking become more difficult, maintaining oral hygiene with swabs can help. These swabs are often provided by the hospice or usually can be found at a local pharmacy. Mouth care can provide an immense amount of comfort, it can be cool/warm, have water or other liquid such as juice for taste, depending on preference. This is very often refreshing and soothing, especially when oral intake of food completely stops.

Pain and symptom management: Managing pain and discomfort through medication is another critical aspect. This will be monitored by your hospice team and often includes narcotics and other medications that are recommended to be on hand if they are needed. Most hospices have a "comfort kit" or list of comfort medications that they recommend, and they will obtain prescriptions for these medications and have them delivered to the individual's house.

Medications often include:

- Morphine/Roxanol for pain and breathing distress.
- Lorazepam/Ativan is used for anxiety and shortness of breath
- Hyoscyamine/Levsin or atropine drops are used to help dry up secretions and congestion.
- Haldol/Haloperidol is used for intense restlessness, intractable hiccups, and sometimes to help with shortness of breath.
- Tylenol/acetaminophen suppositories for fever and pain if the person is not able to swallow.
- Bisacodyl for the bowels as narcotics and other things cause constipation, which can be very painful and uncomfortable if not managed appropriately.

I like to provide a kind of 'comfort statement' as sometimes people struggle with having these medications in their homes. "It is far better to have it and not need it than to need it and not have it."

If there is a pain or breathing crisis, the hospice team does not have any tools to help these symptoms. They will provide a lock box and a designated storage place for safety.

A personal experience: I cannot stress enough how important it is to have this kit on hand. In my practice as a nurse, it has actually only happened to me once, and I am sure you can guess the scenario before I begin to explain. In hospice, we often tell people we are their new '911' and to call us with everything, and we will come and help them with the tools that we have in place.

I had a patient who went into respiratory distress very suddenly and without warning; a diagnosis of lung cancer. With her disease progressing and not responding to treatment, she made the decision to stay at home with hospice care for the duration of her illness. She did not want to go back to the hospital and had chosen this for herself on her advanced directive form. Without morphine in the house, there was nothing that we could do to help palliate her symptoms and keep her home. She was transported to the hospital for management, and guess what they gave her? On her discharge, she consented to having the kit in the house after the extremely scary experience of not being able to breathe and nothing to help at home, where she wanted to be.

Comfort medications can be essential in maintaining symptoms at home and allowing for improved management and quality of life while staying at home.

Medication Management

- Ensure medications are given on schedule.
- Monitor for side effects or changes in behavior after administering medication.
- Keep a log of medications administered, including time and dosage and why you gave it. Was it scheduled or as needed to take care of symptoms?

Pain and Discomfort

- Watch for non-verbal signs of pain, such as grimacing, moaning, or restlessness.
- FLACC Pain Scale (Face, Legs, Activity, Cry, Consolability)

This scale is commonly used for children or patients unable to communicate their pain. Each category is scored from 0 to 2, with the total score ranging from 0 (no pain) to 10 (severe pain).

CATEGORY	0	1	2
Breathing	Normal	Occasional laboured breathing, short periods of hyperventilation	Noisy, laboured breathing, long periods of hyperventilation, Cheyne-Stokes respiration
Negative Vocalization	None	Occasional moan or groan, low-level speech with negative content	Repeated, troubled calling out, loud moaning or crying
Facial Expression	Smiling or inexpressive	Occasional laboured breathing, short periods of hyperventilation	Facial grimacing
Body Language	Relaxed	Tense, distressed, pacing, fidgeting	Rigid, fists clenched, knees pulled up, pulling or pushing away
Consolability	No need to console	Distracted or reassured by voice or touch	Unable to be consoled, distracted, or reassured

FLACC Pain Scale

Total FLACC Score Interpretation:

- **0:** Relaxed and comfortable
- **1-3:** Mild discomfort
- **4-6:** Moderate pain
- **7-10:** Severe pain or discomfort

This tool is usually designed to assess pain in patients with advanced dementia, who may not be able to verbalize their pain. Like the FLACC, each category is scored from 0 to 2, with a total score ranging from 0 to 10.

PAINAD (Pain Assessment in Advanced Dementia)

CATEGORY	0	1	2
Face	No expression or smile	Occasional grimace or frown	Frequent frown, clenched jaw, quivering chin
Legs	Normal position, relaxed	Uneasy, restless, tense	Kicking or legs drawn up
Activity	Lying quietly, normal movement	Squirming, shifting, tense	Arched, rigid, or jerking
Cry	No crying	Moans or whimpers, occasional complaint	Crying steadily, screaming, or sobbing
Consolability	Content, relaxed	Reassured by occasional touching, hugging, or being talked to	Difficult to console or comfort

PAINAD

Total PAINAD Score Interpretation

- 0-1: Minimal or no pain
- 2-4: Mild pain
- 5-7: Moderate pain
- 8-10: Severe pain

Communicate with the healthcare team to adjust pain management as needed. Use prescribed pain relief methods, including medication and non-medication approaches (e.g., soothing touch, quiet environment, repositioning, imagery).

Hygiene and Incontinence Care

- Assist with toileting and incontinence care regularly to

maintain cleanliness and prevent infections. Treat infections if possible.
- Ensure proper bathing and skin care to prevent rashes or irritation.
- Use absorbent pads and diapers as needed to manage incontinence.

Signs of Deterioration

- Be aware of changes in breathing patterns, consciousness, or responsiveness.
- Look for signs of discomfort or distress that may indicate a need for medical intervention.
- Keep in close communication with hospice or healthcare providers about any significant changes.

Environmental Comfort

- Create a calming atmosphere with soft lighting, comfortable bedding, and familiar surroundings.
- Play soothing music or other comforting sounds.
- Keep the environment quiet and peaceful to reduce anxiety.

Emotional Well-being

- Provide reassurance through gentle touch, calming words, and being present.
- Watch for signs of anxiety or distress and offer comfort interventions and presence accordingly.
- Encourage expressions of emotions, whether through talking, writing, or other means.

- Talk to social workers and spiritual supporters to help you process during this time.

Supplies and Equipment Considerations

To ensure that you can provide the best care possible at home, you may need some essential equipment. A hospital bed can make repositioning easier and more comfortable for the individual. Other items, like urinals or bedpans, incontinent care supplies, and extra linens, are important for managing incontinence and maintaining hygiene. Some of these items are provided by a professional service such as hospice; get a list of what they can and cannot provide. It's also essential to have a reliable way to obtain and dispose of medications and medical supplies that are not needed.

While it can be challenging, this is an opportunity to provide care that is full of love and compassion. Remember, you don't have to do it alone. Hospice, palliative care, and end-of-life professionals are there to support you every step of the way, ensuring that you have the right tools and can provide the best care possible.

Self-Care Checklists for Caregivers

Physical Self-Care

- Rest and sleep: Aim for at least 7-8 hours of sleep each night, or take short naps when possible.
- Eat nutritious meals: Ensure you're eating balanced, regular meals, even when things are hectic.
- Stay hydrated: Drink enough water throughout the day.
- Exercise: Take short walks, stretch, or do light exercises to release tension. Exercising too much can actually

put a lot of stress on your body, causing cortisol levels —the hormone linked to stress—to rise, which isn't helpful if you are already under severe emotional strain. When cortisol stays high from overdoing it, it can mess with your sleep, lower your immune system, and make it harder to recover. Staying active is important, but it's just as essential to give yourself time to rest instead of wearing yourself down.
- Take breaks: Step away for a few minutes to rest, even if it's just to sit in silence or step outside for fresh air.
- Avoid over-reliance on caffeine, power drinks, or alcohol: Try not to use these as coping mechanisms.

Emotional & Mental Self-Care

- Acknowledge your feelings: It's okay to feel sadness, frustration, or guilt. Allow yourself to feel without judgment.
- Talk to someone: Share your thoughts with a trusted friend, family member, or support group.
- Seek professional support: Consider speaking with a counselor or therapist if you need emotional/mental guidance.
- Set healthy boundaries: Recognize your limits and don't be afraid to ask for help when you need it.
- Practice mindfulness or meditation: Even a few minutes of deep breathing or meditation can help center your mind and body.
- Do something you enjoy: Whether it's listening to music, reading, or watching a favorite show, carve out time for small pleasures.
- Stay informed but not overwhelmed: Understand the situation, but don't overwhelm yourself with too much medical information.

- Write in a journal: Express your thoughts or frustrations through writing.
- Engage in activities that calm your mind: This could be puzzles, art, knitting, or another relaxing hobby.
- Give yourself permission to step back: Taking time for yourself doesn't mean you're neglecting your loved one.

Social Self-Care

- Reach out to others: Stay connected with friends, family, or support groups, even if it's just for brief chats.
- Ask for help: Be clear and direct with family or friends about the support you need, whether it's running errands or offering a break.
- Accept support: Allow others to assist you without feeling guilty or inadequate.

Spiritual Self-Care

- Engage in prayer, reflection, or meditation: If spirituality is part of your life, find comfort through your practices.
- Connect with nature: Spend a few moments outdoors to ground yourself and find peace.
- Talk to a spiritual advisor: Seek guidance or comfort from clergy, chaplains, or a spiritual mentor if that aligns with your beliefs.

Practical Self-Care

- Organize your caregiving tasks: Make a list of what needs to be done and delegate where possible.

- Create a schedule: Structure your day to include caregiving duties, other work, and breaks for yourself.
- Prepare for emergencies: Have medical and family contacts on speed dial and medications ready, so you're not caught off guard.
- Plan for your own time: Block out regular times for yourself in your calendar, just as you would for caregiving tasks.

Respite

The Medicare hospice benefit allows for a 5-day respite during each benefit period of hospice care. This allows caregivers to set up time where caregiving is provided elsewhere or by hired help. This is underutilized in helping caregivers to maintain the level of care they want to provide.

Remember

- Be kind to yourself: Caregiving can be emotionally and physically exhausting. It's okay to feel overwhelmed at times.
- Celebrate small victories: Acknowledge the little things you accomplish each day.
- Don't forget to breathe deeply; it helps your nervous system. I have compiled a whole section on how breathing exercises can help you in Chapter 12.

Chapter 4

Medications, Comfort Interventions, and Natural Remedies

"The art of living well and the art of dying well are one."

— Epicurus

In the throes of end-of-life care, the focus often naturally shifts from trying to treat an illness to making sure they're comfortable and at peace as much as possible. Medications and other comfort interventions become essential tools in helping manage symptoms and ensuring there is no unnecessary pain or distress. It can be hard to witness a loved one go through pain and panic during these final stages. It may also feel very overwhelming to stay on top of all the different medications needed. Understanding their purpose, however, will make this challenge a bit easier. And don't forget to reach out to your hospice/end-of-life team for questions and guidance.

We've spoken briefly about a "comfort kit"—sometimes called an emergency kit or hospice kit. This is a collection of medications specifically chosen to help manage the most common symptoms that might arise as a person nears the end. Having this kit on hand can help avoid unnecessary trips to the hospital and ensure your loved one stays comfortable. As the body weakens, symptoms like pain, anxiety, and nausea can become more intense and can be remedied at home. It's a core belief in hospice care that no one should have to endure pain when it comes to dying. Relieving pain isn't just about physical comfort—it's about assisting your loved one to spend their final days in as much comfort as possible.

Medications in a Bit More Depth

Morphine or Roxanol: One of the most used medications in the final stages. It's incredibly effective at managing severe pain and shortness of breath, providing relief when your loved one needs it most. Many people struggle with the use of narcotics for this purpose and feel that they are hastening the process; this is false. While the thought of using morphine might seem intimidating, in the hands of a hospice team, it's a powerful way to bring comfort and palliation to the individual.

Levsin/Hyoscyamine and Atropine Drops: These are often used to manage secretions in the throat that can build up and cause a rattling or "percolating," wet sounds whilst breathing. This can be distressing to hear, but these medications help to dry up mucus and make breathing easier and more relaxed. Remember, this is often more difficult to listen to than it is for the person themselves. Check if they have a relaxed face and body.

Haldol/Haloperidol: Used to manage extreme agitation, hallucinations that are distressing, nausea, or vomiting. It helps calm the mind and body, which can make a huge difference in your loved one's end stages. It has also been used for shortness of breath and intractable hiccups, as it has relaxing properties.

Lorazepam/Ativan: Used to relieve anxiety, helping to ease emotional and physical distress. Lorazepam is also used for nausea and shortness of breath.

Tylenol/Acetaminophen Suppositories: Come into play if your loved one has mild to moderate pain or fever and can no longer take medications by mouth.

Additional Medication Options

- **Stool Softeners:** Medications like docusate sodium (Colace) can help soften the stool, making it easier to pass.
- **Laxatives:** Senna (a natural stimulant laxative) can be effective in stimulating bowel movements. Bisacodyl (Dulcolax) or polyethylene glycol (Miralax) can also be prescribed to help with regular bowel movements.
- **Suppositories or Enemas:** In cases of more severe constipation, glycerin suppositories or enemas may be recommended to relieve discomfort and help clear the bowels.
- **Methylnaltrexone (Relistor):** This is a medication specifically used for opioid-induced constipation and can be helpful in end-of-life care for patients on strong pain medications.

Natural Remedies

- **Hydration:** Ensure the person is staying hydrated. Warm liquids like herbal teas or water can help stimulate bowel movements.
- **Prune Juice or Prunes:** These are a gentle, natural laxative that can help relieve constipation. Prune juice is often used to soften stools and promote bowel movement.

- **Fiber-Rich Foods:** Foods like oats, fruits (especially apples, pears, and berries), and vegetables can help regulate bowel movements. However, in some cases, high-fiber foods might not be suitable if the person is very immobile or eating very little, so consult with a doctor first.
- **Gentle Movement:** If possible, even light activity like walking or moving in bed can help stimulate bowel function. For bedridden individuals, gentle leg movements or range-of-motion exercises can be beneficial.
- **Abdominal Massage:** Lightly massaging the lower abdomen in a clockwise direction can help stimulate bowel movement. A healthcare provider can show the appropriate technique.

Fever and Pain Interventions

For natural cooling, apply cool cloths to the forehead, groin, and armpit/axillary area, and remove covers. Apply cold or heat to painful areas. Elevate edematous or swollen areas to assist fluid drainage.

Breathing Comfort

Using a fan directly can assist people to feel less breathless. It is important to recognize that this is not effective in all cases, and very often interventions such as inhaled or nebulized medication and oxygen may be needed for breathing comfort.

At some point, the hospice team may suggest stopping medications that aren't really needed or working anymore. Things like blood pressure meds, cholesterol drugs, or even vitamins might not be as important because the focus is now all on comfort. Letting go of these medications can make things simpler—fewer side effects, fewer pills to deal with, and less confusion from managing polypharmacy. This can ease the load, both for your loved one and for you as their caregiver.

It's a good idea to keep medications pre-filled and organized so when the time comes to make changes, you're ready without any extra stress. It's a small step, but it can make a big difference in ensuring your loved one's comfort. The hospice nurse will be keeping an eye on medications during each visit, helping with refills, pre-filling syringes, and organizing meds so as to take some of that responsibility off your shoulders.

Checklist for Medicating a Loved One at End-of-Life

- When giving liquid medications such as Morphine and Lorazepam, make sure that mouth care has been provided. This is the quickest route of administration other than IV. The mucosa of the mouth must be moist to allow medication to be absorbed. Therefore, frequent mouth care should be provided, and medications should be given prior to this.
- Atropine, Morphine, and Lorazepam do NOT need to be swallowed. They can be ordered in liquid form and are absorbed through the mucous membrane of the cheek under the tongue. This way, they work faster for symptom relief.
- To alleviate the bad taste of morphine or other medications, suggest products with ginger in them, such as ginger ale or crystallized ginger, to help neutralize the taste.
- Extended-release medications cannot be crushed. When crushed, it is no longer extended release and will give the entire dose in one application.
- Immediate-release medications can usually be crushed or scored. With Lorazepam and Levsin in pill

form, these can be crushed and made into a paste to be placed in the cheek to absorb.

Understand the Purpose of Each Medication

Know why each medication is prescribed (e.g., pain relief, anxiety reduction, managing secretions). Ask the hospice team to explain the benefits and potential side effects.

Monitor for Pain and Discomfort

- Regularly check for signs of pain, such as facial expressions, restlessness, or moaning.
- Administer pain medications like morphine as prescribed to keep your loved one comfortable.

Manage Anxiety and Restlessness

- Use medications like Lorazepam to help alleviate anxiety and promote relaxation.
- Keep the environment calm and comforting to support the medication's effects.

Control Secretions

Administer Levsin or Atropine drops to manage throat secretions and prevent the "death rattle." Monitor breathing and adjust medication as needed for comfort.

Ensure Proper Use of Medications for Nausea and Agitation

- Use Haloperidol (Haldol) as directed to control nausea or agitation.
- Observe for any side effects and communicate with the hospice team for adjustments.

Maintain Bowel Regularity

- Follow the prescribed bowel regimen to prevent constipation, especially when using narcotics.
- Ensure regular bowel movements to avoid discomfort and complications.

Stay Organized

- Pre-fill medications as much as possible to ensure quick and easy access when needed.
- Keep a log of when and how much medication has been administered.

Discontinue Unnecessary Medications

- Discuss with the hospice team which medications are no longer needed (e.g., blood pressure meds).
- Understand the rationale for stopping certain medications to focus on comfort.

Communicate with the Hospice Team

- Keep in regular contact with the hospice team for guidance and support.
- Report any changes in symptoms or concerns about medication effects immediately.
- Inform them when you need more comfort medications for refill.

Watch for Side Effects

- Be aware of the potential side effects of each medication and how to manage them.
- Adjust medication under the guidance of the hospice team if side effects occur.

Respect Your Loved One's Comfort and Dignity

- Prioritize your loved one's comfort over all else.
- Ensure that medications are administered gently and with respect for their dignity.

10 Natural Remedies for End-of-Life Patients

1. Lavender Essential Oil

- **Uses:** Lavender is often used for its calming and soothing properties. It can help reduce anxiety, promote relaxation, and improve sleep quality.
- **Application:** It can be used in aromatherapy (diffused in the room), applied topically (diluted with a carrier oil), or added to a warm bath.

2. Chamomile Tea

- **Uses:** Chamomile is well-known for its relaxing effects and can help curb anxiety, insomnia, and digestive discomfort. It can also provide gentle pain relief and support restful sleep.
- **Application:** Drinking chamomile tea or using chamomile in a compress for its anti-inflammatory and soothing properties.

3. Peppermint Oil

- **Uses:** Peppermint oil can help relieve nausea, headaches, and digestive issues, which are common discomforts. It may also provide a cooling sensation that can soothe the skin.
- **Application:** It can be inhaled, applied topically

(diluted), or used in a cold compress for headaches and nausea relief.

4. Ginger

- **Uses:** Ginger is effective in reducing nausea and vomiting. It can also help with digestion and may have mild pain-relieving properties.
- **Application:** Ginger can be consumed as a tea, in small food quantities, or as a compress for its warming and soothing effects.

5. Frankincense

- **Uses:** Frankincense has been traditionally used for its spiritual and grounding properties. It can help with anxiety, respiratory issues, and create a peaceful atmosphere.
- **Application:** It can be used in aromatherapy, applied topically (diluted), or used as a fragrance in burners during meditation or prayer.

6. Aloe Vera

- **Uses:** Aloe vera is known for its skin-soothing properties. It can be particularly useful for soothing bedsores, dry skin, or any other skin irritations.
- **Application:** Aloe vera gel can be applied directly to the skin to heal and moisturize.

7. Lemon Balm

- **Uses:** Lemon balm has calming effects and is often used to reduce stress, anxiety, and promote restful sleep. It also has mild pain-relieving properties.

- **Application:** It can be consumed as a tea, used in aromatherapy, or applied topically as a balm or lotion.

8. Valerian Root

- **Uses:** Valerian root is a strong herbal remedy for anxiety, restlessness, and insomnia. It can help with sleep disturbances and provide a calming effect.
- **Application:** It can be taken as a tea, tincture, or in capsule form.

9. Eucalyptus Oil

- **Uses:** Eucalyptus is often used to ease breathing difficulties and provide respiratory support. It has decongestant properties when there is a cough and can ease chest discomfort.
- **Application:** It can be used in a diffuser, inhaled through steam, or applied topically (diluted).

10. Turmeric

- **Uses:** Turmeric is known for its anti-inflammatory and antioxidant properties. It can help manage pain and inflammation and support overall well-being.
- **Application:** Turmeric can be added to food, taken as a supplement, or used in warm milk (often called "golden milk").

Important Considerations

- Always consult with a healthcare provider before using natural remedies, especially in end-of-life care, as they may interact with medications or specific conditions.

- Dosages should be carefully considered, and remedies should be tailored to the individual's needs and preferences.
- The individual's comfort and quality of life should be the primary focus.

Chapter 5

Celebrations of Life, Funeral Services, and Planning

"Death smiles at us all, and all we can do is smile back."

— Marcus Aurelius

Life can be honored in many ways. When life comes to an end and a soul has left this world, most faith traditions, cultures, and rituals have various ways to care for and prepare the physical body and the spirit that is within. It gives us time to start grieving, to be together, and to express our love for this person we loved and the life they lived. These rituals allow families and loved ones to express their love and respect for the soul that is now gone from them forever. Traditional funeral services are still a common choice, as they offer a structured way to come together and say our goodbyes. A funeral service often includes a wake or visitation, a formal ceremony, and the burial or cremation. It provides space for reflection, remembrance, and support.

But not everyone wants to go down that route. Some of us prefer a celebration of life, with gatherings held in various settings, like at a favorite park, in someone's home, or at a location further afield that holds a special meaning. This allows for a more personalized, creative last rite, with opportunities to include music, stories, and other activities that reflect the person's personality and passions.

There are various alternative options for those of us seeking something different. Green burials are becoming very popular as the eco-friendly choice of being "planted" as a tree appeals to those who wish to leave a positive environmental impact.

Some opt for memorial services without the body present or even virtual gatherings. These can all be meaningful ways to honor a life, especially when family and friends are dispersed across the globe. The key is to find an approach that feels authentic in the way in which someone (we) lived.

Burial, Cremation, and Alternative Options

The choice of either a burial, a cremation, or an alternative option is worth discussing and planning way ahead of time.

Burial provides a physical place where loved ones can visit and pay their respects. Whether it's a family plot, a single grave, or a mausoleum, the act of burial in a graveyard or cemetery provides a sense of permanence and connection. Some choose burial because of religious or cultural beliefs, while others simply find comfort in having a dedicated plot to be laid to rest.

Cremation offers a different flexibility. The ashes can be kept in an urn, scattered in a meaningful location, or transformed into keepsakes like jewelry. Many find this choice comforting, as it provides the opportunity to keep a part of their loved one close or to return them to a place they held dear.

Cultural and Religious Practices

These play a significant role in end-of-life decisions. Understanding these practices is essential to ensuring the farewell is respectful, meaningful, and aligned with the person's values. Such cultural practices can vary widely, reflecting the diversity of religions and traditions worldwide.

For many Christians, death is marked with ceremonies that honor the individual while reaffirming faith in eternal life. This may include a wake, a church service, and either burial or cremation. Eulogies, prayers, and hymns celebrate the person's life and provide comfort to those in mourning. In Mexico and other parts of Latin America, families celebrate Día de los Muertos (Day of the Dead) as a vibrant, joyful way to honor ancestors with altars, offerings, and gatherings that blend reverence and festivity.

In Hinduism, cremation is the norm as it is believed fire purifies and helps release the soul for its next journey in the cycle of rebirth. Families often perform sacred rituals, such as sprinkling water from the holy Ganges River on the body and chanting prayers to guide the soul toward liberation. After the cremation, the ashes may be scattered in a sacred river, signifying a return to nature and the divine.

In Islam, the body is gently prepared by washing it with care and wrapping it in simple white cloth, symbolizing humility and equality before God. Burials occur quickly, usually within 24 hours, with the deceased placed on the ground facing Mecca. The community gathers for a prayer service, and family members often engage in ongoing acts of charity or remembrance to honor their loved one.

Jewish traditions emphasize prompt burial, typically within a day, as a sign of respect for the deceased. Afterward, families observe Shiva, a seven-day mourning period where loved ones stay together, reflect on memories, and welcome visitors who offer their condolences. This time of communal mourning helps the family feel supported while processing their loss.

In Buddhism, death is seen as a transition, and rituals often focus on supporting the soul's journey to its next life. Family members may offer food, incense, or prayers, while monks recite sacred texts to bring peace and guidance. In Tibetan Buddhism, readings from the *Bardo Thodol* (Tibetan Book of the Dead) are common, offering direction for the soul during the intermediate state between death and rebirth.

Resources for Funeral Planning

Planning a funeral or celebration of life can feel overwhelming, especially when emotions are high. That's why it's so important to explore available resources and ensure that everything is in place when needed.

Pre-planning services are a good opportunity to make arrangements in advance, covering everything from selecting a funeral home to deciding on the flowers or the type of service. This can reduce stress for everyone involved, and loved ones can then focus on grieving and remembering you rather than worrying about logistics. When choosing a funeral home, consider factors like location, reputation, and the services offered. Pre-planning can lock in today's prices for extra financial peace of mind.

There are many online resources available to guide you through the process. From how to write obituaries to creating digital memorials, these tools can help you plan a service that reflects your wishes and values. Financial planning resources, such as funeral insurance or trusts, can help cover the costs and make certain that your loved ones aren't left with unexpected expenses.

How to write a eulogy:

https://www.memorialstories.com/blogs/memorial-inspiration/how-to-write-a-eulogy

How to write an obituary:

https://prowritingaid.com/how-to-write-an-obituary

Remember that support services are available through community organizations, religious institutions, and grief counseling groups. These resources are great for emotional support, practical advice, and a compassionate network. Bereavement support through hospice usually lasts 13 months. Celebrations of life are often held annually or bi-annually to honor and remember the person who has passed.

Making Final Plans

Planning for death may not be something you want to think about, but doing so can be one of the most compassionate gifts you give yourself and your loved ones. Making these decisions together can help alleviate anxiety and stress when death does occur.

Early planning allows you to choose and create a checklist of things you want, things you don't want, and what you need to take into consideration, such as what funeral home service will be used or if you have other preferences. Sensible questions need to be asked, like: where will a funeral service be held? Are there any rituals that need to be considered? By discussing these details and taking steps now, you can approach the future with a sense of relief, knowing that everything will be in place when the time comes.

Other Considerations for Burial

Choices about what they'll wear, whether the casket will be open or closed, or if there will be a private family viewing become opportunities to honor who they were and bring comfort to those left behind. These moments allow families to reflect on the unique essence of their loved one and create a final tribute that feels right and meaningful.

Burial Clothing

Choosing what your loved one will wear for their burial is a tender act of love. For some, this might mean selecting a formal outfit that reflects their dignity, such as a favorite suit, dress, or traditional religious attire. For others, it could mean something more personal, like their coziest sweater or a casual outfit that truly embodies who they were.

Many families choose to include sentimental items—perhaps a scarf they always wore, a piece of jewelry that held special meaning, or even a handwritten note tucked into their hands. These decisions are not about perfection; they're about creating a sense of familiarity and closure.

Open or Closed Casket

Deciding whether to have an open or closed casket is a profoundly personal choice. An open casket offers a chance for loved ones to see the person one last time, to feel the tangible reality of their goodbye. It can be a moment of peace, allowing mourners to be close to their loved one and say what's in their hearts.

On the other hand, a closed casket may feel more fitting for families who want to focus on memories of their loved one as they were in life, as viewing the body would be too painful. Whatever the decision, it should be guided by what feels most respectful of the individual being honored.

Private Family Viewing

A private family viewing offers a quiet, sacred space for loved ones to say their goodbyes away from the public eye. In this intimate setting, there's room for raw emotion and personal rituals—perhaps a prayer, a whispered poem, or leaving a gift or cherished keepsake in the casket.

For families who choose a closed casket for the public service, this moment can feel especially meaningful, allowing a final opportunity to say the last goodbye. It's a time to grieve freely, to lean on each other, and to hold space for shared memories and tears.

Chapter 6

Environment and Sensory Considerations

"All you touch and all you see is all your life will ever be."

— Pink Floyd

When we or a loved one is near the end of this life, the spaces around us become so much more than just rooms; they become sanctuaries, sacred places where every detail matters. The environment we create for someone during these precious final moments can be a gentle embrace of familiar sights, sounds, and sensations.

Lighting in the room should be calming as harsh, bright lights can feel clinical and intrusive, like an unwanted visitor. On the other hand, soft, ambient lighting like dimmable lamps or salt rock lamps brings a sense of tranquility. Natural light, where possible, is, of course, best—maybe the soft glow of the morning sun or the golden hue of a late afternoon, reminding us of life's enduring pace and the world's beauty even as someone or we ourselves prepare to leave it. The peace this small environmental consideration can bring is profound.

Sounds in the room should be chosen with great care, like a soundtrack to this final chapter; it matters in the end. Focusing on playing a person's favorite music, movie, TV show, podcast, audiobook, or meditation CD can be very comforting. Even a simple fan noise can bring more serenity. If your loved one enjoyed being at the beach, the sound of waves can be very calming.

However, some may prefer silence or only the gentle rustle of leaves outside or listening to thunderstorms or rain outside the window.

Try to be mindful of other sounds in the immediate vicinity. Keep news programs or violent/disturbing movies or shows out of earshot. Also, remember that any discussions around the patient should be mindful or taken elsewhere. Any heated confrontations need to be taken outside. Even a non-responsive individual can still hear you, even if unable to respond.

Tip: If there is loud equipment such as an oxygen concentrator, consider putting it outside the room to allow for a quieter ambiance.

Touch is another sense that can't be overlooked. Soft blankets and smooth textures can be a great sensory support. Maybe a favorite old sweater or a well-worn quilt—which can bring happy memories of a life well-lived.

Massages and Reiki have also recently been introduced into hospice care as a regular and available holistic practice to ease the symptoms of the dying. Such practitioners bring a different dynamic to the patient through gentle massage. It can also be administered anywhere, be that in bed, a wheelchair, or an armchair.

I myself regularly provided hand massages with lotion, especially for people who were not responsive. It's very soothing and a simple gesture that anyone can manage. Another good area to massage with the thumb is just between the eyes. That area can be very tense, and massaging will often help relieve restlessness.

Scent is powerful, too, in creating a harmonious ambiance. Our sense of smell is deeply linked to our memories and a very individual thing. Try to keep strong and overly chemical scents at bay. Our sense of smell can be heightened at the end of life and typically strong odors and perfumes are often not tolerated well. However, a familiar smell may be welcome, such as fresh fruit or a favorite soap or laundry detergent, or natural scents of certain flowers.

Lastly, think about the space itself and what it holds. Keep it personal and intimate. Photos of loved ones, treasured keepsakes, and meaningful objects. Items that tell stories of love, laughter, and life. The environment in the last moments should be a reflection of the person's preferences and your understanding of it.

Chapter 7

Grief and Bereavement

"Grief is just love with no place to go."

— Jamie Anderson

It is said that grief is a journey. It often begins long before the actual moment of death, and many of us continue to mourn and remember our lost loved ones for a long time after. Grief is not something that just hits you and then goes away. In fact, many people will tell you that it never really leaves; you just learn to live with it differently.

Grieving is not a static experience, despite the well-known five "stages" in which grief typically manifests itself: denial, anger, bargaining, depression, and acceptance.

It is important to remember that these stages occur in different sequences for all of us. But knowing them can help us to identify why we feel the way we do or why others grieve differently.

Grieving helps us to heal ourselves from the losses we experience.

It can be especially intense when you're caring for someone and witnessing their decline. In my experience with hospice care, I've seen how grief can take many forms—anticipatory grief is just as real and complex as the grief that comes after someone dies.

It can be devastating, this saying goodbye in small doses, day after day, until we say it for the final time. There can be mixed feelings when someone passes: relief, disbelief, sadness, remorse, anger, and resentment even. Remember that it is okay to feel all these emotions. Allow yourself to experience the moments and let them help guide you to a place where acceptance and peace can manifest.

Here is a wonderful TedTalk on grief and grieving:

https://www.ted.com/talks/david_kessler_how_to_find_meaning_after_loss?subtitle=en

Humans are, however, not the only living beings that grieve. It has been well-researched, and many animals do, too. Crows, magpies, jays, and ravens, for example, hold funerals for their dead members. You may also have heard that elephants literally bury their dead and have special burial grounds where they gather and honor the bones of their deceased.

Whales and dolphins have been known to carry their young with them for weeks, and other members of the school circle around a dead calf. Or dogs that will not move from the grave of their owner. These are all physical manifestations that animals comprehend loss, grief, and honor their dead.

Honoring Personal Choice

As we have discussed previously, personal choices toward the end are paramount. However, it is worth mentioning again, as when we grieve, we can often lose sight of this. One of the greatest gifts we can give to someone nearing the end of their life is the freedom and autonomy to choose how their journey will go.

There are, of course, conditions when this may not be possible, such as with dementia or other circumstances where the person is not able to talk anymore. In this situation, the guidance I can provide is to be brutally honest with that reality and focus on what you know about them. Caregiving in such times can take a huge toll on everyone involved, which is why, as we go through the motions, it is important to draw on the resources that are available to navigate this better.

For Caregivers

Caregivers often burn themselves out in their mission to remain strong for everyone else. This puts them at risk. You've heard the phrase "it takes a village"—and that is true. Without the right support, things can catch up fast and become overwhelming and exhausting. Caregiver burnout is a real thing, as is compassion fatigue. Remind yourself not to feel guilty, and admit when you are exhausted, tired, or struggling. This is the best course of self-care and a must! You can't take care of anyone if you don't take care of yourself. Think of the plane/oxygen mask example. Who does the flight attendant tell to put the mask on first?

Build in sensible time-outs here and there: take a walk, make a cup of tea, have a long shower, or take a car ride. Find time to let yourself cry as well as laugh, and deliberately find these moments of release and joy. Under strained circumstances and emotional turmoil, everyone understands that you will need to regroup, breathe a bit deeper, and take a few minutes to rest. We are all only human, and there is no need to punish yourself with guilt trips. It will help you get through the hard things still to come.

The Role of Hospice Social Workers and Chaplains

Hospice social workers and chaplains are instrumental in helping us to get through such intense times, when we naturally need more emotional, mental, and spiritual support.

I've been lucky to work with some of these incredible professionals, and their ability to offer compassionate help is such a blessing. These special people are not only there for the dying but also for the family and caregivers. Having their involvement and being able to have their support is invaluable and can be a great comfort.

Hospice Social Workers

The hospice social worker is a licensed medical social worker. They provide support to both patients and families who find themselves in the midst of an end-of-life situation. They provide emotional and bereavement support and act as an advocate. They assist in coordinating care needs and services and help procure other care resources so families can navigate their care requirements. They also provide assistance in finding financial and other support that may be available within the community.

These professionals are here to listen and sit with us in our sadness, processing all aspects of the end of life. They can be a catalyst and encourage us to have tough conversations, like discussing advance directives. Hospice social workers can support complicated grief situations, such as those involving children or complicated family dynamics. It can be very healing to voice our fears and emotions to someone empathetic. These wonderful people really make a difference. When hospice is involved, they typically follow families for 13 months to provide bereavement and grief support if needed.

Chaplains

Whether or not you are religious, chaplain support tends to be non-denominational. In other words, they support all faiths and spiritual practices. Chaplains are here to provide support ranging from praying with us to providing end-of-life blessings or organizing spiritual practices, such as bespoke funeral services. This support can mean very different things to different people. Chaplains can bring peace, decrease fear, and assist in finding closure. They will sit without judgment, ensuring a safe space for what we need to process.

Navigating the Complexity of Emotions

We all need to realize that grief is always messy. One second, we're okay; the next, a small thing can trigger and totally overwhelm us and unleash an avalanche of fear, sadness, guilt, and anger. Some days, we'll manage just fine; other days, the whole world seems to want to swallow us whole. The important thing is to allow all emotions to flow. Suppressing them has never been a good strategy because in our vulnerabilities we can also find grace.

I've seen families avoid talking about the reality of death because it's too painful, and while that's understandable, it can also create distance. Having those difficult conversations can actually bring us closer together. Togetherness can be a great healing agent, but we must be brave and help each other through it.

Rebecca A. Brewer, RN BSN CHPN

The Mental Health Aspect of Grief

It may surprise you to hear what goes on in our brains when we grieve. It may also help to clarify the confusion and agony somewhat and emphasize our collective humanness when such tragedies occur.

If grief feels unbearable or there are persistent symptoms of depression or anxiety, it's important to seek professional help. Grief counseling, therapy, or support groups can make a world of difference in helping our brains and hearts heal.

Hidden Stages of Grief and How to Cope

Anticipatory Grief

When we're aware that a loved one is nearing the end, the mourning of their absence often starts already while they're still alive.

How to Cope:

- Acknowledging our feelings: Recognizing that feeling sadness, anger, or guilt before a loss is natural. Giving ourselves permission to feel these emotions without judgment.
- Creating meaningful moments: Spending quality time with our loved one, reminiscing, saying what needs to be said, or simply being present.
- Seeking support: Talking to others who are going through similar experiences can be comforting. Hospice counselors, support groups, or even trusted friends can help us process the rollercoaster of emotions.

Feeling Disoriented

The Last Season

When faced with the loss of a loved one, life can start to feel unreal or disjointed—a dream-like reality that just doesn't seem real. This disorientation may involve feeling like we're living in a haze, disconnected from daily routines or people.

How to Cope:

- Grounding helps: Focusing on small, manageable tasks to bring ourselves back to the present moment. Surround yourself with environments and people who bring comfort and peace.
- Self-care: Grief takes a toll on the mind and body, so prioritizing rest, hydration, and activities that bring happiness is strongly encouraged.
- Talking it out: Sharing our sense of confusion or surreal feelings with a friend or counselor can help buffer the experience.

Helplessness

Feeling helpless and adrift is common when we realize there's little we can do to stop decline and death.

How to Cope:

- Controlling what we can: Even small gestures, like providing comfort through touch or words, can make a big difference.
- Reframing our role: Recognize that presence and support are powerful acts of love, even when we can't "fix" the situation.
- Seeking practical support: Asking for help with caregiving tasks or emotional support can reduce feelings of loneliness and helplessness.

Emotional Numbness

When overwhelmed by the situation, we may feel emotionally numb and disconnected from reality.

How to Cope:

- Giving ourselves grace: Emotional numbness is a temporary response to overwhelming feelings.
- Talking when ready: Speaking with a loved one or professional can help us gently tap into those emotions.
- Engaging in small activities: Doing familiar tasks can help create a sense of normalcy.

Resentment

We may experience resentment toward the situation, a loved one, or even ourselves for being placed in this position.

How to Cope:

- Recognizing it's normal: Feeling resentment doesn't mean we love someone any less.
- Practicing self-compassion: Remind yourself that these feelings stem from sadness.
- Venting safely: Utilize the hospice team and other supports to express these feelings constructively.

Hope for Release

There may come a point where we begin to hope for our loved one's peaceful release from all the suffering.

How to Cope:

- Understanding it's normal: Wishing for the end of suffering is a compassionate response.

- Focusing on comfort: Ensuring the last experience is peaceful and as pain-free as possible.
- Leaning into support: Hospice teams and counselors can help us process these conflicting feelings.

Fear of Life Without Them

As the loss approaches, fear about what life will look like without a loved one may become overwhelming.

How to Cope:

- One day at a time: Focus on today and slowly ease back into routines.
- Asking for help: Reach out to family, friends, or professionals.
- Building a support system: Keep close the people who can offer support during and after the loss.

Mixed Relief and Sadness

Once the loss occurs, many of us will experience a mix of relief and sadness.

How to Cope:

- Giving ourselves permission to feel: Allow both emotions to coexist without guilt.
- Sharing it: Express mixed emotions with someone who understands.

Further Tips and Resources

Before seeking the support of a grief counselor, consider the following:

- Identifying your needs: Reflect on the specific aspects of your grief and what you hope to achieve through counseling.
- Researching credentials: Ensure the counselor is licensed and experienced in grief counseling.
- Understanding therapeutic approaches: Familiarize yourself with counseling methods to find one that resonates with you.
- Assessing comfort level: Feeling at ease with your counselor fosters open communication.

For more guidance, the American Counseling Association offers resources on finding a grief counselor: American Counseling Association - Grief Counseling.

Chapter 8

Making Things Easier

"Accepting help is its own kind of strength."

— Kiera Cass

Accepting Help and Finding Resources During End-of-Life Care

Caring for someone at the end of life is a time filled with so many emotions, love, exhaustion, and sometimes a heavy sense of responsibility. But we don't have to do it all alone. Accepting help and using resources can lighten the load, allowing us to focus on those precious moments with our loved ones. One of the main points is allowing help. On that note, remember to…

Let People Help You. When we care for someone, it's natural to feel like we should handle everything ourselves. But caregiving is a big job, and there's no shame in letting others lend a hand. Remember, accepting help doesn't mean we're not strong—it means we're human.

Letting People Know How They Can Help: Sometimes, people want to help but aren't sure what to do. If someone offers, don't be afraid to suggest specific tasks. Whether it's cooking a meal, running errands, or simply sitting with them while we rest, even small gestures can mean so much.

Creating a Network of Support: We might be surprised how many people would be willing to help if they knew how. A good idea is to set up a network where family and friends can sign up to assist with different tasks. This way, the responsibility doesn't fall on just one person, and we'll have more time to spend with our loved ones without feeling overwhelmed.

Reaching Out to Support Groups: Connecting with other people who are going through similar experiences can provide comfort. Support groups—whether online or in person—offer a safe space to share our feelings and pick up practical tips from others who understand exactly what we're going through.

Seek Help When You Need It: Taking care of someone at the end of their life is hard, both physically and emotionally. It's okay to need help. Recognizing when we're stretched too thin and asking for support can make all the difference in keeping ourselves well enough to care for them. We talked about some of these already, but here they are in summary:

Look into Respite Care Services: Respite care is like a reset button. Hospice organizations often offer these services, where a professional caregiver takes over for a few hours or even a whole day. This gives us time to rest, recharge, and care for our needs. It's not selfish but essential.

Consider Counseling or Therapy: Caring for someone can stir up all kinds of emotions. Talking to a therapist can help us work through feelings of grief, guilt, or even anger. There are also grief counselors who specialize in end-of-life situations, offering support both during and after the experience.

Use Hospice and Palliative Care Resources: Hospice and palliative care teams provide not only medical support but also emotional and spiritual care. Many include social workers, chaplains, and other counselors who can guide us and our loved ones through this journey. We should never hesitate to ask them for help—they're there for all of us, patients, family and caregivers. They can also be instrumental in allocating other services that might be needed in the community such as private care and complex grief counseling.

Tools and Resources for Caregivers

There are lots of resources out there that can make day-to-day caregiving more manageable. From organizing schedules to making sure we're eating well, these tools can help us stay on top of things.

Scheduling and Coordination Tools

Lotsa Helping Hnds: This is a free online tool where you can set up a community of support. You can post requests for specific tasks—like meal prep, running errands, or just sitting with your loved one and people can sign up to help. It's an easy way to keep everyone organized and involved.

CaringBridge: Not only can you coordinate care here, but you can also share updates about your loved one's condition. This can save you the stress of having to give the same updates to multiple people. It keeps everyone in the loop while letting you focus on what really matters.

Shared Calendars (like Google Calendar): Sometimes, the simplest tools are the most effective. A shared calendar helps you coordinate doctor visits, medication schedules, and visits from family and friends. It's a small way to stay organized when things feel hectic.

Meal Planning and Delivery Support

Meal Train: Meal Train makes it easy for friends and family to sign up to bring meals, ensuring that you're well-fed even on days when you're too busy to think about cooking. You can set it up so meals are dropped off at certain times, giving you one less thing to worry about.

Take Them a Meal: Similar to Meal Train, this site allows people to sign up for meal deliveries, and you can specify dietary needs or preferences. It's another way for people to help in a way that directly supports your well-being.

Grocery Delivery Services (Instacart, Amazon, Hello Fresh): If cooking isn't an option, grocery delivery services can save you time and energy. You can order online and have essentials delivered right to your door, freeing you up to focus on your loved one.

Medication and Health Management Tools

CareZone: This app is incredibly helpful for tracking medications, symptoms, and appointments. You can also store important medical information here, making it easy to stay organized and informed.

Medisafe: With Medisafe, you'll get reminders for medications and other health-related tasks. It's especially helpful if your loved one has a complex medication schedule, giving you one less thing to remember.

Respite Care Services

National Respite Network: This network can help you find respite care providers in your area, whether you need a few hours or a full day. Taking a break is essential for your well-being.

ARCH National Respite Locator: This service helps connect you with respite care options, offering short-term relief when you need it most. Sometimes, just knowing there's a backup can help you breathe a little easier.

Respite through the hospice benefit: This is a benefit of hospice care which allows for a 5 day respite care stay, usually in a facility such as a nursing home or other inpatient setting such as a hospice home. This benefit makes it possible for caregivers to take a break, while ensuring loved ones are cared for.

Remember to use your resources. Talk to your family and friends and accept help. You are not alone. Accepting help and sharing the load can make a challenging journey a little bit lighter. This is important work, and it's okay to reach out and let others be there for us as well.

Creating Boundaries

Sometimes, too much help is simply too much. Very often, people want to support us as much as they can, and at times, this onslaught of kindness can feel overwhelming. To some, this can mean staying with you all day or for hours at a time or even coming every day. Don't be afraid to limit visiting times or to decline help when you just don't want to have visitors that day. Creating a schedule and limiting visits to certain days or times (30 minutes or less) is usually a good idea and, of course, adjustable to whatever is acceptable to you. Sometimes, it is helpful to use online applications such as Meal Train and cancel someone if needed. Even a simple sign on your door indicating 'no visits today' is perfectly okay.

Chapter 9

Considering Pets and Animals

Animals are such agreeable friends. They ask no questions; they pass no criticism.

— George Eliot

Many of us have the joy of having pets that make our lives complete. Suffice it to say that they, too, are affected by lost loved ones and may react in many different ways. It is natural to worry about those animals who are left behind, including beloved pets. They have been there, offering companionship and unconditional love through life's ups and downs. Not only at the very end, but during decline too, they feel what is happening. It's important to make space for them too and ensure they're provided for.

Animal Behaviors

Pets are intuitive, especially toward the humans they are closest to. Their love is unconditional. They experience loss and grief, too. In many instances, their behavior can be confusing; some pets want to be close to their dying person, and others want to stay away.

Conversely, especially cats and dogs will often want to be in bed with their person and snuggle up close to their body. Or they may linger very close by, such as under their bed, refusing to leave the room, or even resist going outside. Their eating and bathroom habits may change, too, as a further expression of their stress.

Assessing a Pet's Needs

Every pet is unique, and understanding their specific needs can help guide you in making the right decisions. Consider their daily routines, favorite foods, and potential medical needs. This is a time to think about what makes them feel comfortable and safe.

Involving the Vet

A vet can provide guidance on handling transitions and potential behavioral changes and give us tips for easing any stress a pet may feel. They may also be able to recommend local resources or support networks if we need help finding a new home for a pet. Some pets are prone to infections such as urinary tract infections or may have other difficulties that require a vet's assessment. If possible, compile essential pet information so it is in order and readily available. This would include vaccinations and yearly testing for heartworm and tick-borne diseases and other essential documentation.

Preparing a Pet Care Plan

A pet care plan can serve as a detailed guide for anyone who may care for our animals. Include information about their diet, any medications they take, and other routines. If they have certain fears or anxieties, be sure to note these as well. If the pet needs planning for after their person's passing, perhaps consider including provisions for the pet in a will. By planning ahead, we can alleviate potential financial burdens and ensure beloved animals receive the care they deserve.

Identifying a Caretaker

There might be a need to find a loving home if their owner has passed, unless there is a family member or friend who might take on this responsibility. This should be a conversation held well ahead of time to try and make the transition easier when the time comes. If it is a family pet, we might consider asking someone to foster the pet if we are struggling to make sure their needs are met, and have them back when we are ready. If there is a need to rehome them, choosing the right new owner to care for a pet can bring immense peace of mind. My advice is, take time to discuss this with trusted family members, friends, or neighbors who share a genuine bond with your pet. Ideally, choose someone familiar who really has the time, the right set-up, and the love to give.

Should family or friends be unable to help, consider speaking with local animal shelters or rescue groups. Many organizations offer rehoming services or can assist in finding a foster family. Remember, you're not alone, and there are compassionate people willing to ensure your pet's well-being. There are options for a designated person you can name in your will, and funds can also be allocated to them for whatever a pet may need in the future.

Rebecca A. Brewer, RN BSN CHPN

Considering an Unlikely Wish

It is also possible for a pet owner to put in their will that they want their pet to be euthanized if they pass away, but it's not always as straightforward as it sounds. Whether this kind of request is honored depends on local laws, ethical concerns, and the people responsible for carrying out the will.

The Legal Side of Things

Legally, pets are considered property in most places, so technically, an owner can make decisions about what happens to them after they're gone. However, asking for a pet to be euthanized just because the owner has died can raise some serious red flags. Many animal welfare laws are in place to protect pets from unnecessary harm, and putting down a healthy, happy animal simply because their owner isn't around anymore might not hold up in court. The executor of the will, the person responsible for making sure the owner's wishes are carried out, could also refuse to follow through if they feel the request is unethical or could lead to legal trouble.

The Vet's Perspective

Veterinarians play a big role here, too. Most vets take their responsibility to animals seriously and won't euthanize a pet unless it's absolutely necessary for the pet's health or well-being. If they're faced with a perfectly healthy animal, they might refuse to do it, regardless of what the will says.

The Emotional and Ethical Dilemma

This kind of request can be tough for everyone involved. Pets are more than property—they're living beings with emotions and the ability to adapt to new situations. Asking for them to be euthanized might feel like the right way to protect them from uncertainty, but for many, it feels unfair to the pet, especially if they could go on to live a full and happy life with someone else.

Thankfully, there are better options. Most pet owners who love their animals deeply want to make sure they're cared for after they're gone. That's why many people make plans to rehome their pets or set up funds for their care.

Better Alternatives

I already listed many better alternatives, and if you're worried about what will happen to a pet, here are three things you can do to make sure they're safe:

- Choose a caretaker
- Set up a pet trust
- Work with a shelter or rescue

Emotional Well-Being for Pets: Transitioning to a New Home

Pets can sense changes, and they may feel very anxious during transitions. To ease this, we can make sure to provide familiar items, like their favorite toys, blankets, or even an item of clothing. Comforting smells and objects can help them feel secure in an uncertain or new environment. If possible, introduce your pet to new caretakers gradually. Spending time together before the transition can create a sense of trust and familiarity, helping to make the change as smooth as possible.

Legacy of Love: Keeping a Connection

For many, pets are family. Knowing the animal is happy and well can bring comfort to you that you've made a good decision for the well-being of a beloved animal. You can stay in touch via FaceTime or arrange regular visits to keep the connection alive.

Rebecca A. Brewer, RN BSN CHPN

The Many Ways Animals Grieve

We already covered elephants, birds and whale behaviour. Here are some other startling examples from the animal kingdom.

Primates such as chimpanzees, gorillas, and other primates also show signs of grieving. They may groom the bodies of deceased family members, avoid the area where the dead body lies for some time, or display signs of real distress. Chimpanzee mothers have been observed carrying their deceased infants for days, showing reluctance to let go.

Cats are creatures of habit, and losing a beloved human disrupts their world in profound ways. You might notice they're eating less or refuse food altogether, a sign that they're struggling. Their behavior often shifts—they may cry out loudly as if searching for their person or, conversely, retreat into silence. Some cats cling to you more than ever, seeking comfort in your presence, while others wander the house, checking familiar places as though their human might still be there.

Dogs are emotional and expressive by nature, so when they lose a loved one, it's often easy to see their sorrow. They can lose interest in their favorite activities, become lethargic, and skip meals. Some will search tirelessly, sniffing at clothing, lingering by doors, or curling up in spots where their person used to sit. Their eyes, filled with longing, tell a story of heartbreak that words never could. There are also numerous accounts of dogs that would not leave the grave site of their owner for days after the funeral.

Birds like crows or ravens have some of the most remarkable grief behavior observed. When a crow dies, other crows often gather around the deceased. These gatherings can involve dozens of crows, and they may vocalize loudly as if calling out or expressing distress. This behavior has been described as a "crow funeral," where crows will stand vigil, sometimes for an extended period, before moving on. Researchers believe that these gatherings may serve multiple purposes, including mourning and learning about potential dangers that may have led to the death.

Crows and ravens are known for their problem-solving skills and learning behaviors. When they encounter a deceased member of their group, they often approach cautiously and observe the situation as if trying to understand what happened. They can remember faces and places associated with danger, which is why some researchers believe that these "funerals" also help crows and ravens learn about threats to avoid in the future.

Both crows and ravens form strong bonds with their mates and other members of their flock. If a mate or a close companion dies, the surviving bird may show signs of distress, such as becoming more subdued or vocalizing in ways that are interpreted as expressions of sadness or loss.

Ritualistic Behaviors

Ravens have also been observed engaging in what appears to be ritualistic behavior around the dead. They may be seen poking at or nudging the body as if trying to elicit a response. Or they may bring small tokens, such as sticks or leaves, to the deceased bird, which some interpret as a form of ritual.

These grieving behaviors are significant because they highlight not only the emotional depth of animals but also their advanced cognitive abilities and emotional capacities.

Chapter 10

The Last Season

To everything there is a season. A time for every purpose under heaven; A time to be born, a time to die. Everything has its time. A time to heal, a time to break down. A time to build up and a time to weep. A time to laugh and a time to mourn.

— Ecclesiastes 3:1-8

Facing the end of life is something none of us can ever fully prepare for, and yet, when the time comes, we find ourselves searching for ways to bring comfort, dignity, and peace to those final moments. These times in our lives are often a kaleidoscope of emotions—sorrow, love, anger, confusion, and sometimes even a quiet sense of relief. By understanding what we can do to ease this last chapter—whether through personal rituals or cultural traditions—we can also help others to make this transition as easy as possible.

The Power of Being Present

Don't be afraid to talk, even if the person dying or you yourself are not able to respond. The human voice carries great healing and soothing powers, as does touch. Touch, soft speech, and just being in the room can bring the needed peace. Be fully present and don't be afraid. Use these final moments to really reaffirm your bond and love.

Being Absent

Sometimes, you will not be able to be present when someone dies. People can pass away when they are alone in the room. Sometimes, it may even feel like that was the thing they were waiting for. Don't feel bad or guilty about this. This, too, is out of our control. It depends on who the person was during their lifetime. A strong person may not want anyone to see them this way.

Cultural and Spiritual Traditions at the Time of Passing

I already spoke about the different cultures and their own beautiful ways of guiding someone through the last moments. Let's take a closer look at some of these rituals:

Buddhist Practices: In Buddhism, those final moments are viewed as profoundly significant, with the belief that they can influence the soul's journey onward. Family members or monks may gather to chant mantras, filling the space with peace and clarity. It's a time for mindfulness and acceptance, allowing the person to transition with a calm mind and an open heart.

Islamic Prayers: For Muslims, saying the Shahada—a declaration of faith—is a vital part of the final moments. Family members may quietly repeat these words, helping to center their loved one's focus on their faith and their connection with Allah. They may also turn the person to face Mecca, wrapping them in the spiritual comfort of their beliefs as they prepare to leave.

Catholic Last Rites: In Catholicism, a priest may perform the Anointing of the Sick, offering prayers, forgiveness, and anointing with holy oil. This sacrament brings spiritual peace and healing, as family members may gather in prayer by their loved one's side, united in faith and love as they support their journey into the next life.

Hindu Mantras and Rituals: In Hindu tradition, family members often recite sacred mantras, and they might offer a few drops of holy water from the Ganges River. These practices serve as blessings, guiding the soul and helping it transition with purification and a deep sense of spiritual connection.

Jewish Recitations: For those of the Jewish faith, the Shema is often recited as death approaches, affirming the unity of God. Family members may also read psalms, creating a sense of unity and focusing on honoring the sacredness of their loved one's passage while drawing strength from their shared faith.

For some, like in certain Native American traditions, the belief is that the spirit will return to the Earth or be reunited with ancestors. In these final moments, families may sing or offer prayers, surrounding their loved ones with a sense of unity, continuity, and peace as they cross over. And there are many, many more cultural rituals globally.

The Last Breath: A Profound Transition

That final breath often feels like the closing of a beautiful chapter that we can never read again. It may be followed by a deep stillness, where time seems to pause, and everyone present takes in the weight of the moment. It's common for families to hold each other close, cry together, or say a final prayer, even share funny stories and memories. Some may choose to simply sit in silence.

Although grief may begin to settle in, these moments often carry a powerful sense of love and connection that lingers, helping to cushion the first steps into what needs to be done.

Ways to Remember

There are so many ways to remember someone that go beyond the traditional. When we're looking to honor a loved one, finding a way that feels truly unique to them and our relationship can bring solace. Here are some creative and meaningful ways to keep their memory alive, celebrating who they were in a way that feels truly special:

Send Off a Biodegradable Balloon or Lantern

An eco-friendly balloon or paper lantern release can be a beautiful way to say goodbye. You can write little notes, memories, or wishes, then watch them float up together. It's a simple yet touching way to let go, and doing it at dusk can make for a really memorable moment.

Make a Time Capsule of Memories

You could gather photos, letters, and small keepsakes that remind you of your loved one and tuck them into a time capsule. Plan to open it on a special anniversary or save it for future generations. It's a way to capture those memories and keep them safe for years to come.

Create a Signature Scent Just for Them

Smells can instantly bring back memories. Consider working with a perfumer to design a scent inspired by them—whether it's based on a flower they loved or a smell that reminds you of their favorite place. Wearing it or simply having it nearby can evoke a comforting sense of closeness.

Get a Memorial Tattoo with Their Handwriting or a Special Symbol

Tattoos can be deeply personal and a great way to carry someone with you. Think about incorporating their handwriting, a favorite quote, or a symbol that represents them. It's like having a piece of them with you always, in a form that's uniquely yours.

Name a Star After Them

You can register a star in their name and receive a certificate with its location. On clear nights, you can look up at the sky, find their star, and feel a little closer to them. It's a simple yet beautiful way to create a lasting tribute that's out there in the universe.

Host a "Living Memorial" Event Based on Their Passions

If they loved art, food, or music, why not throw a celebration that's all about what they enjoyed? You could organize a group painting class, cook up their favorite dishes, or even have a jam session. It's a great way to honor them in a way that reflects their personality and brings people together.

Have Their Ashes Pressed into a Vinyl Record with Favorite Songs

Some companies can mix ashes into a vinyl record. You could choose songs that were meaningful to them or even record personal messages and have those included. It's a unique keepsake that combines music and memory in a way you can actually listen to.

Design a Custom Puzzle or Game About Their Life

For those who loved a good game night, think about creating a puzzle or board game that tells their story. You can include fun facts, photos, and inside jokes. It's an interactive way to share memories, especially if they were known for their sense of fun and laughter.

Create an Ocean Memorial Reef from Their Ashes

If they loved the ocean, consider having their ashes mixed into a reef ball and placed in the sea. It helps restore marine habitats and creates a lasting memorial that supports the environment. You could even make a trip out and visit the site on anniversaries.

Create a Gemstone from Their Ashes

Memorial diamonds or other gems can be made from ashes, turning them into a stunning piece of jewelry. It's a way to have something beautiful and lasting that symbolizes their presence and the enduring impact they had on your life.

Commission a Personal Art Piece or Portrait

You could have an artist create something that reflects their spirit—a portrait, a symbolic piece, or even something abstract that captures their essence. Hang it somewhere special, and it'll be a constant reminder of who they were and the love you shared.

Dedicate a Day to Acts of Kindness in Their Honor

If they were known for their generosity, why not honor them with a day dedicated to acts of kindness? Friends and family can do things like volunteering, donating, or simply helping someone out. It's a beautiful way to spread their kindness and keep their legacy alive in a way that's positive and meaningful.

Turn Their Social Media into a Digital Memorial

Social media profiles can be transformed into digital tributes where friends and family share photos, memories, and stories. It's like a living scrapbook that everyone can contribute to, making it a virtual space to visit and reflect whenever you need to.

Send Around a "Traveling Journal" of Memories

Start a journal with a few stories about them, and then pass it to others to add their own memories. When it's filled up, you can bring everyone together to share the stories. It's a wonderful way to remember them and celebrate the joy they brought to everyone's lives.

Make a Memorial Quilt from Their Clothes

If they had favorite shirts, scarves, or even old blankets, consider making a quilt from them. Each square can represent a different memory or moment, creating something warm and tangible that wraps you in comfort and love whenever you need it.

Choosing something that feels right and reflects our loved one's unique spirit can make all the difference. These creative ways to remember them aren't just tributes; they're ways to keep their memory alive in our daily lives. Whatever we choose, may it bring peace and remind us of the beautiful times we shared.

The After

We may get swallowed up by grief and the feeling of our loss. Grief is much like a tide that comes crashing over you at any minute and threatens to take you out with it, never to return to the sure you knew.

We may find ourselves asking, what comes now? What comes after their death? Life may feel so different.

Allow yourself to feel the loss and feel the sadness fully, but don't live continuously there. We have to remind ourselves that life goes on. That it's ok to laugh and find joy, even though we may feel like a smile will never touch our lips again, but it will.

The tears will seize, and the sadness we may experience in the months and years to come will eventually fade and turn into acceptance.

What comes after is trying to live life as fully as possible and create our own extraordinary journey until it is time for our last season.

Chapter 11

Changes at the End of Life

"In the end, it's not the years in your life that count. It's the life in your years."

— Abraham Lincoln

Here we will discuss changes that may be noticeable months, days, weeks, hours, and minutes before death. Being aware of what to expect, such as social withdrawal, decreased appetite, and increased sleep, helps us to understand these changes as they emerge. A decline in health is often gradual and difficult for caregivers to witness. Therefore, a lot of reassurance needs to be provided. It is always a good idea for caregivers to discuss what they are capable of and willing to do (feeding, hydrating, other activities, etc.) and where other support may have to be called in.

Dehydration is a natural process that occurs when the body starts to actively decline and get ready to transition. This is a very difficult process for most to witness. We feed and give people fluids and medicine to help them feel better. However, as the body declines, its functions start to slow down, and there is no longer the same need for food and water. A good rule to follow is to pay attention to what the individual wants and to see if it's safe. If food or fluids are refused, let them. If they want a sip or taste of something, that's okay too. If there is swallowing difficulty, or the person is not able to swallow or be upright to take, drink, or eat, do not try to force them. This can cause aspiration of fluid or food into the lungs, which can be very uncomfortable. Good and frequent mouth care, use of lip salve, and mouth swabs can be very helpful during this phase to keep the mouth moist and provide comfort. You can find these swabs at most pharmacies, and they are usually provided with hospice care. These swabs can be dipped in any liquid, including water, juices, or anything that might taste good. They can also be used to clean the mouth.

Bear in mind that dehydration is a normal part of dying. It does not hurt, and in many cases, it helps make the transition easier.

Eating changes are another difficult topic that can stir up many emotions. As someone approaches the final stage, their appetite often fades, and they may no longer want to eat much or nothing at all. This can be incredibly hard to watch for family and loved ones, especially since we're so used to equating food with caring, nourishment, and love. But just like dehydration, a decreased desire to eat is a natural part of the dying process. Forcing this may cause more harm than good, leading to nausea or vomiting, causing distress and often pneumonia, or further congestion and shortness of breath.

At this stage, there may be minimal intake, and that's okay. Usually, small, soft foods like pudding, applesauce, or something similar are good options if they desire to eat. Sometimes, tasting something they once loved can bring pleasure even if they can't eat much or need to spit it out after tasting. It is important not to put too much pressure on eating at this time; by the same token, if there are requests for specific things, try to honor this.

Changes in Consciousness and Alertness

As the body winds down, changes in consciousness may occur and can be unsettling for both the individual and their loved ones. Moments of lucidity may feel fleeting, and they may appear as though they are caught between worlds. For those witnessing this, it can be a deeply emotional experience, as the person might suddenly seem engaged and then drift away again. Cherishing these moments of presence, however brief, and offering consistent, gentle affirmations of love and safety can create a serene atmosphere, even as the boundaries between wakefulness and sleep blur.

There may be periods of delirium and confusion as the brain activity declines. Handle this with patience and understanding, meeting the person where they are to provide them with reassurance.

Physical Weakness and Fatigue

The body gradually prioritizes its energy for essential functions, leaving little for physical movement. This profound weakness can also feel like a loss of independence for the individual, which may evoke frustration or sadness. It is crucial for caregivers to approach this with sensitivity, preserving dignity by offering help in a way that feels collaborative rather than intrusive. Small acts of support, such as lifting a hand to their lips for a drink or adjusting their pillow, can communicate respect in these intimate moments. Also, remember to talk to the individual if possible and include them in decision-making and discussion about their care needs.

Changes in Skin Color and Temperature

The coolness and discoloration of the skin can serve as a visible reminder of the body's waning strength, often signaling that the end is near. These changes can evoke feelings of grief for loved ones, as they represent the physical transformation of someone they cherish. Expressing your love in a tactile and nurturing way, offering a sense of connection even as the body begins to let go, is a great gift to the dying.

Decreased Urine Output and Bowel Changes

These physiological changes often underscore the gravity of the situation, as they reflect the body's gradual cessation of vital functions. For caregivers, addressing these needs can feel like an act of devotion. While these moments may seem purely clinical, they can also be deeply human, providing an opportunity to demonstrate love when words may no longer suffice.

Increased Restlessness or Agitation

This stage often feels like the body and mind are struggling to find peace. For those bearing witness, it can appear as if the person they care for is uncomfortable or distressed. However, this restlessness is often part of the body's natural letting go process. Providing comfort might go beyond physical reassurance—speaking in a calm, grounding tone can remind them they are not alone. These small yet profound gestures not only ease their passage but also allow loved ones to feel that they are contributing to a sense of peace during this difficult time.

Social Withdrawal

As the journey nears its end, withdrawing from social connections is a way for an individual to conserve energy for their transition. Such a withdrawal can be difficult for loved ones to accept, as it may feel like a rejection. However, respecting their need is the best way forward here. Sitting silently by their side, reading softly, or simply holding their hand without expectation can create a sense of closeness even in the absence of words. Social visits and gatherings may not be of interest or may be very short-lived.

Surge of Energy

Unexpected bursts of vitality, however spontaneous, can feel like a precious gift. It is an opportunity for loved ones to share a meaningful moment, whether through laughter, conversation, or fulfilling a simple request, like a favorite meal or song. While the subsequent decline can be heart-wrenching, it helps to view this surge as a natural part of dying, often providing closure and a final expression of connection. Embracing this moment without over-interpreting it allows caregivers to savor its beauty while preparing for the final goodbye.

Changes in Breathing

Breathing changes are one of the most obvious ways we can see that the end is near. We may see our loved one's breathing becoming slower, with long pauses in between. This can be heart-wrenching to listen to—it may even frighten you—but be assured that this is just the body's way of preparing itself for the final act. The most important thing we can do is stay at their side and let them know we're there. Even if they may not be responsive anymore, it will bring them more comfort than you can imagine.

But what can breathing changes near the end really look like?

Cheyne-Stokes Breathing

A more irregular breathing pattern that can emerge; at times speeding up, then suddenly slowing down again. A loved one may stop breathing for a few seconds altogether. Try not to get anxious, and remember that observing and being present is all we can do here.

Pauses in Breathing (Apnea)

In moments where a loved one stops breathing for a while, we can find ourselves holding our own breath. An unsettling feeling for sure, but this, too, is natural. Such apnea can grow longer since the body needs less oxygen.

Shallow or Labored Breathing

It can also occur that breathing becomes strained or shallow. We may even detect that a loved one uses their shoulders or neck muscles to force breathing. Remaining calm is key here. Additionally, with comfort medications put in place, the respiratory system can be soothed and ease the distress.

"Death Rattle"

One of the most challenging things to hear is the gurgling sounds, called the "death rattle." Unpleasant for sure, but usually not uncomfortable for the individual. All it means is that saliva or mucus in the throat can't be cleared properly. This sounds worse than it is, and there are ways we can help an individual, such as with medications and frequent repositioning.

How We Can Handle End-of-Life Breathing Changes

Rule 1: Stay Calm and Reassured

Taking a few deep breaths ourselves can do wonders. Also check out the specific breathing exercises in Chapter 12. If we can remain a calm presence it will have a great impact.

Breathing Easier with Positioning

We can gently raise their head with pillows. This will make breathing a little easier. Sometimes turning a loved one onto their side helps with the gurgling sounds, allowing fluids to drain more naturally.

Managing Secretions (the Rattle)

If needed, we can ask a hospice nurse about medication that can help dry up secretions or use a humidifier to ease breathing. Suctioning can be an option, but often, it's not needed. Small shifts and adjustments can make a great difference.

Just Being There

Sometimes the best thing we can do is simply sit with them. Holding their hand, talking softly, or just sitting in silence. Our presence—our warmth and care—can provide the support needed in those last moments and ease anxieties. Even if a loved one seems unconscious, our touch and voice can still reach them.

Medications for Comfort

If a loved one is struggling and seems uncomfortable, we can ask for help. Morphine is often used when there is a feeling of not getting enough air or pain. It can make a world of difference.

Creating a Calm Environment

We have already touched upon this. Low lighting, gentle music, and a favorite scent can help create a serene final ambiance. We cannot force this situation to change; rather, we need to lean into it, accept it, and ensure the space is as tranquil as possible.

Other physical symptoms that we may see when someone is nearing the end:

- Increased Sleepiness and Fatigue
- Less Responsiveness
- Periods of Confusion or Agitation
- Visions or Hallucinations
- Unconsciousness

More Unusual Behavior in the Last Stages of Life

Hallucinations and Visions

Seeing or speaking to unseen people: It's not uncommon for people at the end of life to report seeing or speaking with deceased loved ones, spiritual beings, or others who aren't physically present. These experiences can be soothing to the person, and they often talk about these encounters with clarity and calmness. While it can be surprising for those around them, it's nothing to worry about.

Vivid dreams or nightmares: Some individuals may experience vivid dreams or nightmares. They might wake up and recount these dreams in detail or seem confused and disoriented by them. Dreams can be intense, and the emotions they evoke can spill over into wakefulness.

Reaching or Picking at the Air

Restless movements: You might notice someone reaching out or picking at the air or their bedclothes. This behavior, sometimes referred to as "air hunger" or "picking," is often a subconscious response to internal changes in the body, and while it may seem strange, it's usually not a sign of distress.

Grasping at invisible objects: Some people may reach out as if trying to grasp something, sometimes repeatedly. This can be a response to hallucinations or simply an involuntary movement. It's often seen in the final days or hours.

Speaking in Metaphors or Symbolic Language

Talking about going home" or "taking a trip": People nearing the end of life often speak in metaphors, saying things like "I'm getting ready to go on a journey" or "It's time for me to go home." This symbolic language can reflect their awareness of the nearing end, even if they don't explicitly acknowledge it. It can also express their readiness or acceptance of dying.

Unusual Focus on Certain Objects or People

Unfinished business: Some may talk about needing to complete tasks or meet with certain people, even if these tasks are impossible or the people are no longer alive. This can be related to a need for closure or reconciliation.

Fixation on a specific person or object: A dying person might fixate on a particular object, repeatedly asking to hold it. This can be a way of seeking comfort or fulfilling an emotional need.

Reliving past events: Some people may seem to revive past events or experiences, speaking to someone as if they are in a different time or place.

Unexplained Emotional Shifts

Sudden calmness or agitation: A person might suddenly become very peaceful, even if they were anxious or restless before. This can sometimes occur shortly before death, as if they have found acceptance. Conversely, some might become agitated or express strong emotions without a clear reason related to physical discomfort, unresolved issues, or spiritual experiences.

Intense need for reassurance: As the end nears, the person might repeatedly ask for reassurance or express fears about being alone, even if loved ones are nearby. Providing a calming presence, holding their hand, and speaking to them can help alleviate these concerns.

Increased Sensitivity to Surroundings

Heightened sensitivity to light or sound: The dying person may become unusually sensitive to light, sound, or touch, reacting strongly to stimuli that wouldn't normally bother them. This can be a result of changes in their senses as the body shuts down.

Desire for specific environmental changes: They might request dimming the lights, playing certain music, or even requesting silence. These preferences can be their way of finding more comfort during their last moments.

While unusual, these behaviors can still show up as a natural part of the dying process. Providing a calm, supportive environment and being nonjudgmental can help greatly. If you're unsure or concerned about any behavior, don't hesitate to contact a healthcare professional or hospice care provider for guidance.

The Final Moment and Beyond

Once death has occurred, it's time to call hospice or the end-of-life team. They will come and assist us in providing a supportive presence and answering questions the family may have. The RN (Registered Nurse) obtains permission from the doctor for the pronouncement of death and provides postmortem care. The nurse will also help destroy medications and narcotics that are no longer needed and provide initial bereavement support. Postmortem care may include bathing and lotion or special rituals and preparing the person to be taken to the funeral home. It is important to be aware of spiritual or cultural practices as to what is done at the time of death.

In some cultures, it is customary to cover the face of the person, while in others, it is exposed for the family to see. There are many variable practices, and we should be mindful of these important details. Family, if they wish, should be included in the postmortem care. Very often, this helps us get closure when providing this final act of love and care.

Chapter 12

The Self-Care Aspect

"Taking care of myself doesn't mean 'me first.' It means 'me too.'"

— L.R. Knost

In all the preparations and emotional turmoil, we often forget to look at ourselves. Real self-care is an important part of this process. One of the best ways to support ourselves is to learn breathing exercises. These can keep us calm and strong and are great allies.

Deep Belly Breathing

When our emotions start running high, everything feels heavy, and we are full of grief and sadness, deep belly breathing can help greatly. It's a simple way to bring ourselves back to the present moment and counterbalance the pain.

- Sit or stand comfortably. If you're sitting beside your loved one, you can do this right there.
- Take a slow, deep breath through your nose, and let your belly rise.
- Then slowly exhale through your mouth, feeling your belly fall.
- Keep repeating this for a few minutes. Focus on that gentle rise and fall. It'll help ease some of the tension, like a little wave of calm washing over you.

4-7-8 Breathing

- Inhale quietly through your nose for 4 counts.
- Hold that breath for 7 counts (don't worry if it feels long—it'll get easier with practice).
- Exhale completely through your mouth for 8 counts, almost like a slow sigh.
- Do this a few times. As you fall into the rhythm, you'll notice your body starting to relax, like you're gently telling your brain, "It's okay to slow down."

Grounding Yourself

- Sit down with your feet flat on the floor or somewhere in nature. Barefoot would be best.
- Take a second to notice the world around you—the chair beneath you, the grass if you are outdoors, the breeze on your skin, the sound of birds.
- Mentally make a list: 5 things you can see, 4 things you can touch, 3 things you can hear, 2 things you can smell, and 1 thing you can taste.
- Allow yourself to reconnect and linger in the present moment. It's a good way of reminding yourself you are safe, and you can handle this.

Box Breathing (Square Breathing)

- Breathe in for 4 counts
- Hold your breath for 4 counts
- Exhale for 4 counts
- Hold again for 4 counts

Mindful Observation

- Pick one thing to focus on—maybe it's the rise and fall of your loved one's chest, the light filtering through the window, or even the texture of the blanket.
- Zero in on that one thing. Notice every detail, no matter how small. How does the blanket feel between your fingers? How does the light shift?

These little mindful moments of hyper-focus help anchor you in the now, reminding you to just be there.

Mantra or Affirmation Breathing

- Combining your breath with calming phrases can also do the trick to curb anxieties.
- Choose a simple phrase like, "I am safe," "I am calm," or "I am fully present."
- As you inhale, silently say the first part—"I am..."
- As you exhale, say the second part—"... calm" or whatever word feels right.

Let the rhythm of your breath and the mantra soothe you. Even in the toughest moments, these small words can bring a surprising amount of peace, like a quiet reminder that you can handle this.

Hand-on-Heart Breathing

- Place your hand on your heart. Feel its warmth on your chest.
- As you breathe in, imagine the air filling the space around your heart.
- When you breathe out, feel your chest soften and release.

Stay here for a few minutes, just breathing and feeling the connection between your hand and your heart. This is about giving yourself some of the love and care you're giving to your loved one.

Progressive Muscle Relaxation

- Tensing the muscles in your toes for 5 seconds, then relax them.
- Do this slowly, moving up your whole body—tense your calves, knees, thighs, stomach, chest, arms, and face, then release each one.
- As you release each muscle group, imagine all the stress leaving your body, like slowly letting go of all the heaviness you've been holding onto.

Self-Compassion Breaks

- When it all gets too overwhelming, acknowledge what's happening out loud: "This is really hard."
- Remind yourself you're not alone—so many people have been there too.
- Give yourself the gift of kindness. Tell yourself something comforting, like "I'm really doing my best

under the circumstances" or "It's okay to be scared; plenty of others have been here too." Just hit pause and acknowledge your feelings. Giving yourself a little love in such a difficult time is not selfish; it's essential.

Visualization

- Close your eyes and picture a place that brings you peace. Maybe it's the beach, a quiet forest, or a cozy corner of your home.
- Take a few deep breaths as you imagine every little detail—how the space feels, the sounds, the colors, the scents, the textures.
- Stay in this place for a few moments, allowing yourself to feel grounded and calm. This little mental escape can give you just the bit of peace you need to keep going.

Additional Resources

The resources below can help you find necessary support and tools for your family notebook or guide, helping to make the process of end-of-life planning as organized, considerate, and compassionate as possible.

General End-of-Life Planning Resources

MyLivingVoice An interactive tool assists patients to create an advance directive to help guide their medical care choices in the event they are unable to.

mylivingvoice.com

National Institute on Aging (NIA): Provides a comprehensive guide on end-of-life planning, including advice on caregiving, advance care planning, and managing finances.

National Institute on Aging

The Conversation Project: Offers tools, resources, and guidance on how to have important conversations about end-of-life wishes and preferences with loved ones.

The Conversation Project

AARP: AARP's end-of-life planning resources cover various aspects, including health care directives, funeral planning, and organizing important documents.

AARP End-of-Life Planning

Hospice Compare

Their web site offers comparisons and scoring of hospice companies throughout the country. They show you quality measures of the care that they provide as well as input from patient family surveys.

Hospice Compare

Funeral Consumers Alliance

Dedicated to protecting the consumer's right to choose a meaningful, dignified, affordable funeral. FCA is a nonprofit organization that offers education, guidance, and advocacy and acts as an advocate for consumers to choose a meaningful, affordable service.

Funeral Consumers Alliance

FUNERALS360

Provides interactive tools and resources for funeral related needs. FUNERALS360 offers resources and interactive tools to help guide you with funeral details. 360 offers planning checklists, memorials, announcements and resources for veterans' funerals. They offer guidance for financial aspects of and paying for funerals.

FUNERALS360

Legal and Financial Planning

American Bar Association: Has resources related to estate planning, advance directives, and other legal documents that might be part of an end-of-life guide.

American Bar Association https://www.americanbar.org/groups/real_property_trust_estate/resources/

National Academy of Elder Law Attorneys (NAELA): Provides guidance on finding an attorney who specializes in elder law and can help with estate planning, wills, and trusts.

NAELA

Everplans: A digital platform that helps organize and store all end-of-life planning documents, from wills and health care directives to funeral plans.

Everplans

Healthcare and Advance Care Planning

National Hospice and Palliative Care Organization (NHPCO): Offers resources on palliative care, hospice care, and advance care planning.

NHPCO

Prepare for Your Care: This site provides step-by-step guidance on how to make medical decisions, fill out advance directives, and communicate wishes to family members.

Rebecca A. Brewer, RN BSN CHPN

Prepare for Your Care

Five Wishes: A popular resource for creating a living will that outlines personal, emotional, and spiritual needs alongside medical preferences.

Five Wishes

Get Palliative Care

This website provides clear, comprehensive palliative care information and resources to patients and families facing serious, complex illness.

getpalliativecare.org

CaringInfo Provides free resources to help people make decisions about end-of-life care and services before a crisis.

nhpco.org/patients-and-caregivers/

Lotsa Helping Hands Lotsa Helping Hands powers online caring communities that help coordinate daily life help during times of medical crisis. Brings together caregivers and volunteers through online communities that organize daily life during times of medical crisis or caregiver burn-out.

lotsahelpinghands.com

info+contactus@lotsahelpinghands.com

Organizing and Documenting Personal Information

Get Your Sh*t Together (GYSH): This resource helps with organizing life's essential information, such as passwords, legal documents, and insurance details.

Get Your Sh*t Together

Cake: Offers tools for end-of-life planning, including checklists, documentation templates, and storage for digital files.

Cake

Quicken WillMaker & Trust: A software program that assists with creating legal documents for wills, trusts, and more.

https://www.willmaker.com/

CareTree

Caretree.me is a centralized, coordinated health record management system for caregivers to utilize when caring for a loved one. You can create an individual profile for the receiving, with personal demographic information, medication lists, important documents such as MOLST and advanced directives, appointment calendars, and more. Caregivers can access free personalized recommendations for their loved one's care.

caretree.me

Grief Counseling and Bereavement Support

GriefShare: A national organization that provides grief support groups and resources for people experiencing loss. Available in all US states and ten other countries internationally.

GriefShare

The Center for Complicated Grief: The Center for Complicated Grief (CCG) offers educational information regarding complicated grief and provides a tool for finding a therapist who is familiar with it.

info@complicatedgrief.columbia.edu

National Alliance for Grieving Children (NAGC): Offers resources to support children and teens coping with the loss of a loved one.

NAGC

Dougy Center: Provides grief resources specifically for children, teens, young adults, and their families.

Dougy Center

Hand to Hold: This nonprofit provides emotional support and resources to help families before, during, and after NICU stays and infant loss. It is a peer-to-peer support, online community. They can helo with hospital resources and hosts a blog and podcasts to help families before, during and after NICU stays and infant loss. Request for assistance can be initiated via telephone or through an online request form.

handtohold.org

Wonders & Worries

Helps children 2-18 cope when a parent faces a serious or life-threatening illness. All services are offered free of charge to anyone and are available in English and Spanish. In-person support groups, individual sessions, and bereavement and parenting support are also available.

info@wondersandworries.org

Phone: 512-298-3607

Digital Tools for Creating a Family Notebook or Journal

Evernote: A note-taking app that can be used to organize and store end-of-life plans, checklists, and personal reflections.

Evernote

Microsoft OneNote: A digital notebook app ideal for creating sections dedicated to different aspects of end-of-life planning and personal memories.

Microsoft OneNote

My Life & Wishes: An online tool that helps document personal wishes, health directives, and important life information in one accessible place.

My Life & Wishes

Holistic Resources

Natural Medicines

An evidence-based foundation that has an unbiased perspective on natural medicines and uses scientific data to provide practical information for clinicians and patients.

naturalmedicines.therapeuticresearch.com

Diya Holistic Life Care

A nonprofit that provides services through the coaching modality on a pro-bono or sliding-scale basis. They help create custom care plans based on individual preferences, interests, and services. Health coaching, nutrition, health care advocacy, holistic cancer coaching & cancer support, end-of-life coaching, death doula, and other esoteric health care resources. The site provides direct services and can connect you to their podcast series and blogs. VA residents are able to access in-person services; otherwise, they can access services virtually anywhere in the US.

diyaholisticlifecare.org

Phone: 646-926-4590

Wishes and Bucket Lists

Dream Foundation Grants wishes to terminally ill adults and their families by offering end-of-life dreams. This experience can be applied for through the online application. Applicants must be a US resident, diagnosed with a life-limiting illness and have a life expectancy of 12 months or less. They must be in a doctor's care at the time the application is completed.

dreamfoundation.org

Phone: 888-437-3267

application@dreamfoundation.org

1528 Chapala Street, Suite 304, Santa Barbara, CA, 93101

First Descents

Provides free outdoor adventures to young adults who are impacted by cancer and other serious conditions. First Descents offers multi-day and week-long programs to frontline healthcare workers and young adults ages 18-39 who are diagnosed with cancer or other serious health conditions after age 15. The website has a Programs Finder tool that can be searched by community, activity, and duration.

firstdescents.org

Phone: 303-945-2490

info@firstdescents.org

3827 Lafayette St. Ste 161, Denver, CO, 80205

Spouse and Parenting Support

Well Spouse Association

Offers numerous types of emotional support options and education resources to address the challenges and unique issues caregivers face when dealing with a sick spouse.

wellspouse.org

Phone: 732-577-8899

Widowed Parent

Supports widowed mothers and fathers with children in the home. At Widowed Parent, parents can find all sorts of tools regarding the grieving process and resources to help them and their children deal with the passing of a spouse/partner or parent. Practical resources, as well as online and in-person support group options, are listed.

widowedparent.org

Wish Upon a Wedding

A volunteer-run organization comprised primarily of wedding professionals who grant free wedding wishes and vow renewals to couples facing serious illness or life-altering health circumstances. Wish Upon a Wedding is a nationwide nonprofit organization which grants weddings and vow renewals to couples facing terminal illness or serious life-altering health circumstances. Applicants must be aged 18 and older, US citizens,

and have a qualifying health status.

wishuponawedding.org

info@wishuponawedding.org

Veterans

VA Caregiver Support Line

This caregiver support line provides assistance and resources to caregivers of veterans. The Veteran's Affairs VA Caregiver Support Line offers training, educational resources, tools to help caregivers, peer support mentoring, and resources to help caregivers optimize the health and well-being of veterans.

caregiver.va.gov

Rebecca A. Brewer, RN BSN CHPN

Phone: 855-260-3274

LGBTQ Resources

SAGE (Services & Advocacy for GLBT Elders)

SAGE is the oldest and largest organization in the US dedicated to improving the lives of LGBTQ+ older adults. They offer advocacy, services, and resources tailored to the unique needs of this community.

https://www.sageusa.org/

National Resource Center on LGBT Aging

Operated by SAGE, this center provides training, technical assistance, and educational resources to support aging services for LGBTQ+ older adults.

https://www.lgbtagingcenter.org/

LGBT National Help Center

This organization offers free and confidential peer support and local resources for LGBTQ+ individuals, including seniors. They provide hotlines and online chat services.

https://lgbthotline.org/

Human Rights Campaign (HRC) – Mental Health Resources, LGBTQ+ Community

HRC offers a compilation of mental health resources, including support for those facing end-of-life issues.

https://www.hrc.org/resources/mental-health-resources-in-the-lgbtq-community

Hospice Foundation of America – LGBT Resources

Provides information and resources on hospice and palliative care tailored for the LGBTQ+ community.

https://hospicefoundation.org/lgbt-resources/

GLMA: Health Professionals Advancing LGBTQ Equality

A national organization of healthcare professionals advocating for LGBTQ+ health equity, offering resources and directories to locate LGBTQ+-friendly healthcare providers.

https://glma.org/

American Psychological Association (APA) – LGBTQ Resources and Publications

APA provides a range of publications and resources addressing the psychological aspects of aging and end-of-life care for LGBTQ+ individuals.

https://www.apa.org/pi/lgbt/resources/

National Hospice and Palliative Care Organization (NHPCO) – LGBTQ+ Resource Guide

NHPCO offers a comprehensive guide to assist healthcare providers in delivering inclusive end-of-life care to LGBTQ+ patients.

https://www.nhpco.org/wp-content/uploads/LGBTQx_Resource_Guide.pdf

www.ingramcontent.com/pod-product-compliance
Lightning Source LLC
Chambersburg PA
CBHW050310230526
45471CB00005B/2108